Neurosurgical Procedures - Innovative Approaches

Edited by Alba Scerrati and Pasquale De Bonis

Published in London, United Kingdom

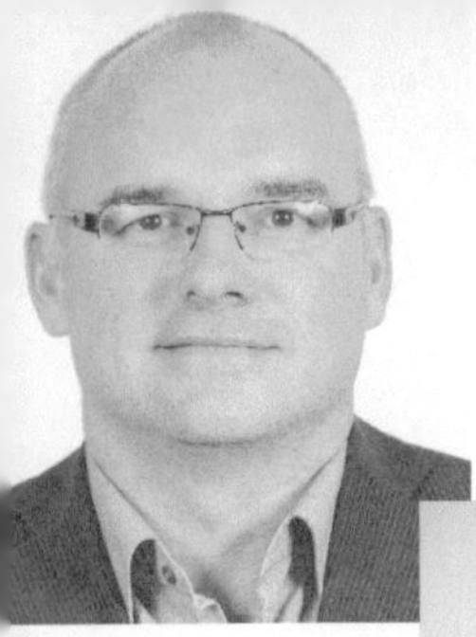
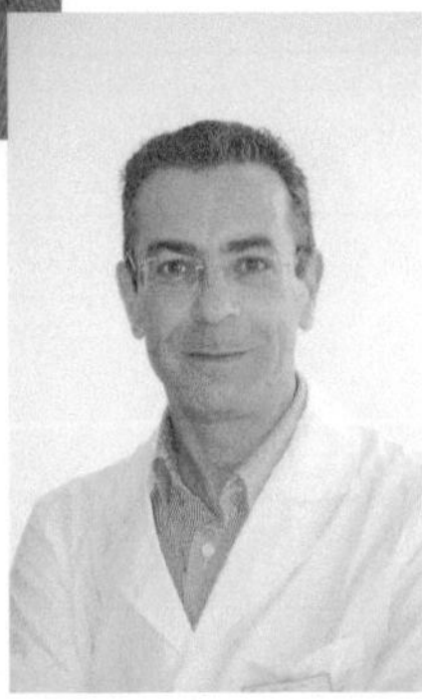
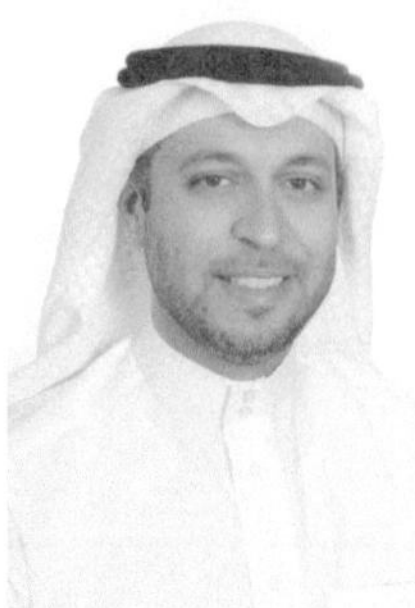
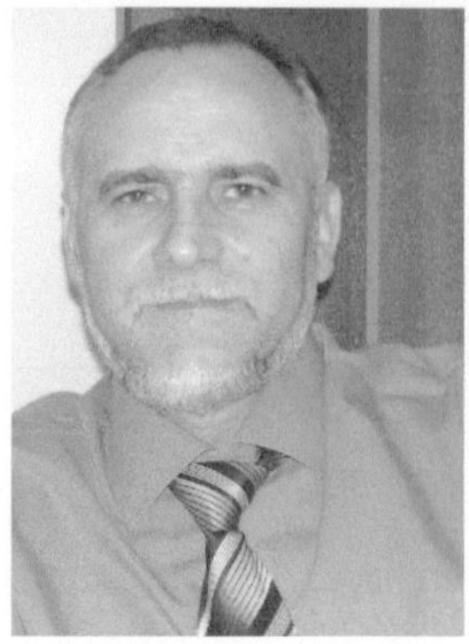
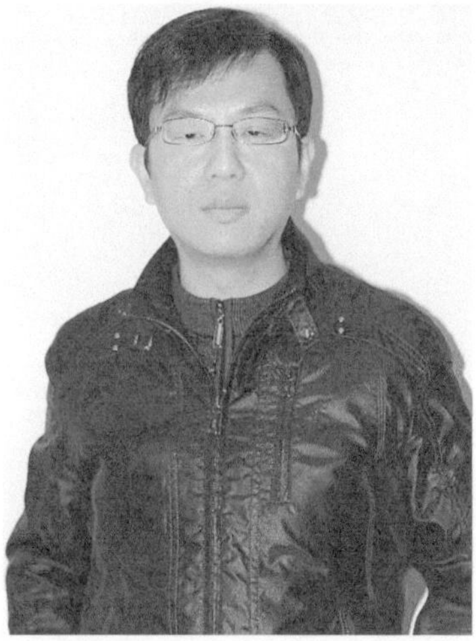
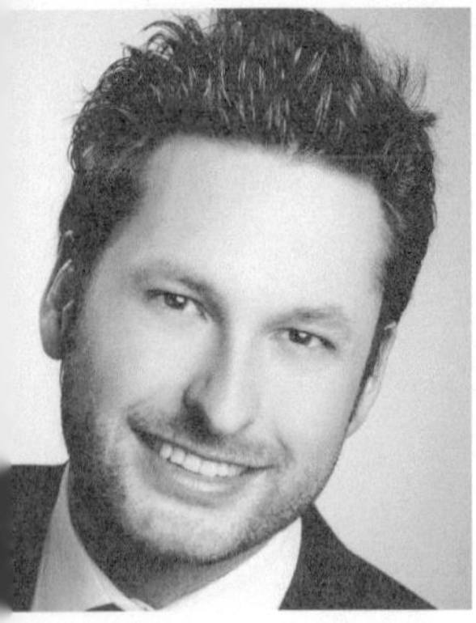
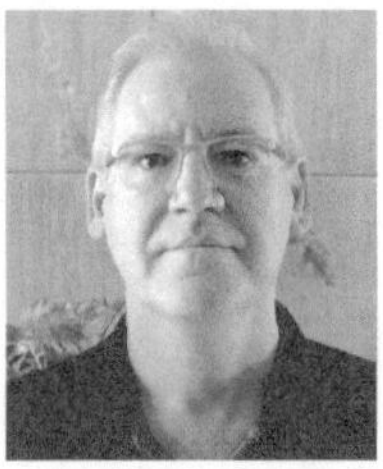

IntechOpen

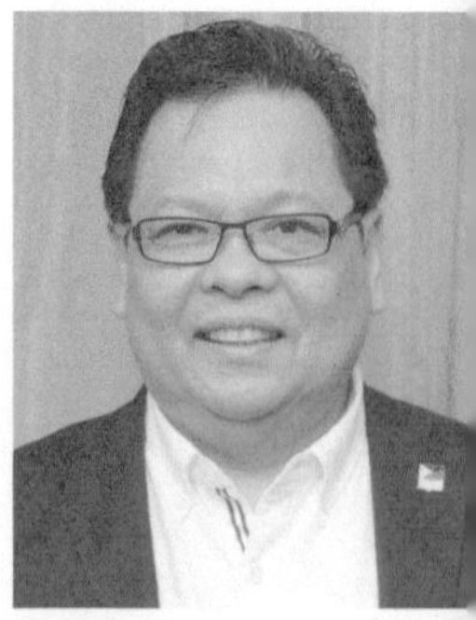
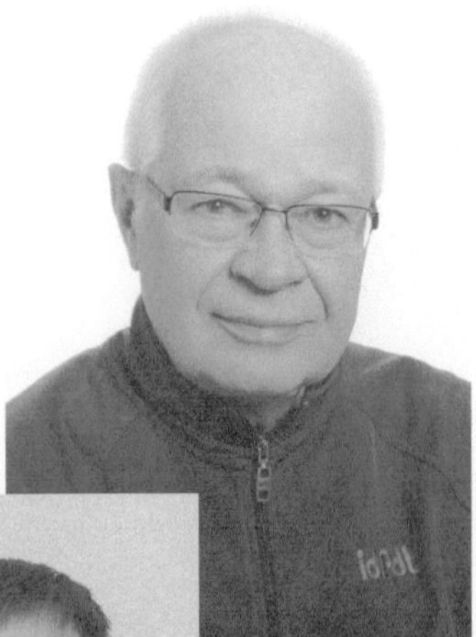
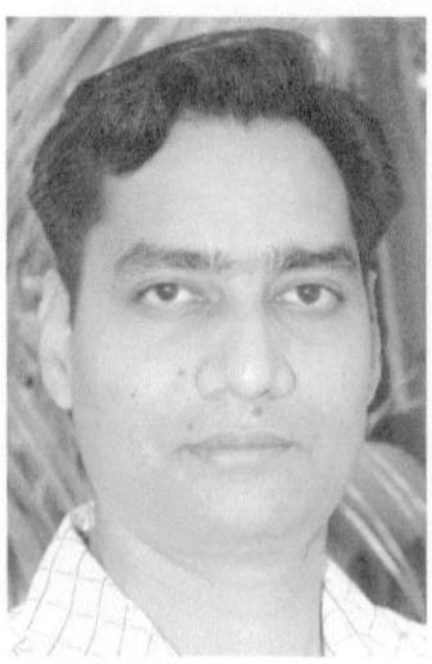
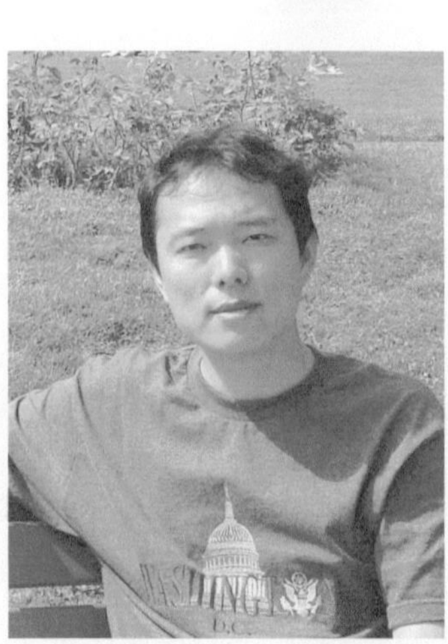
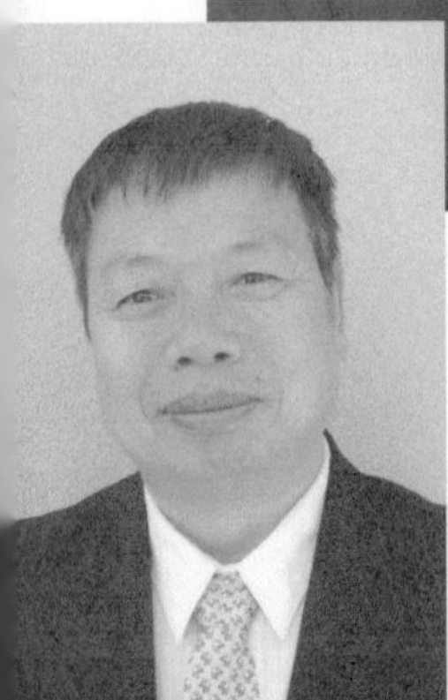
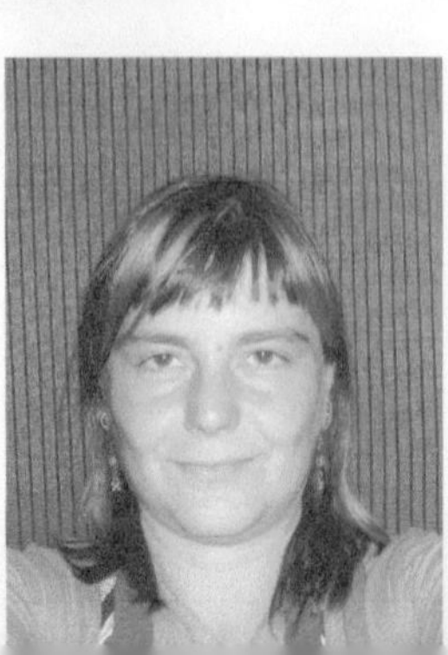

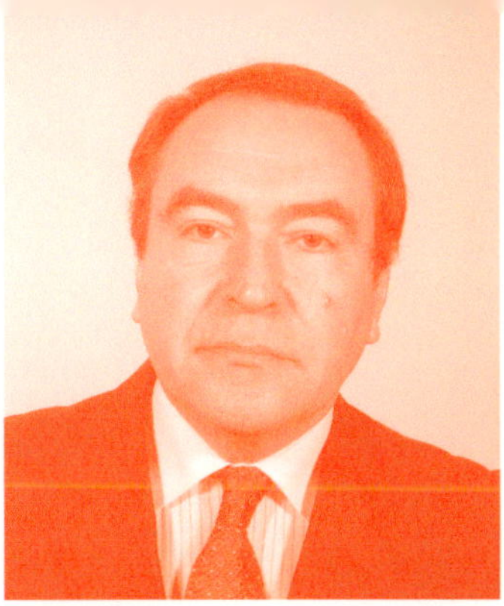
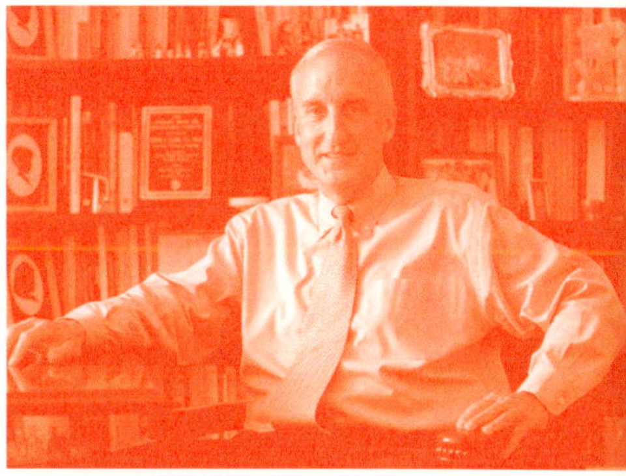
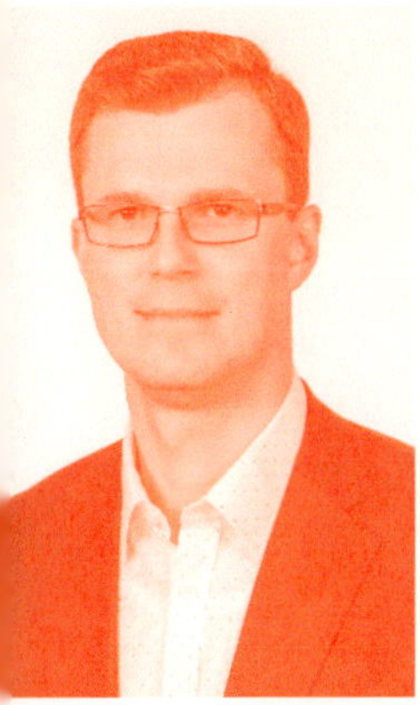
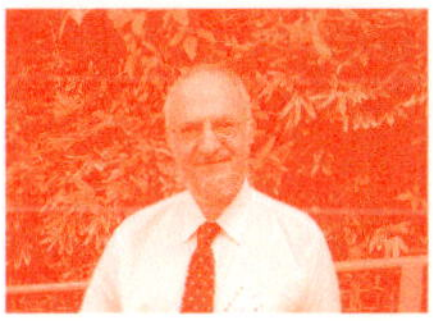
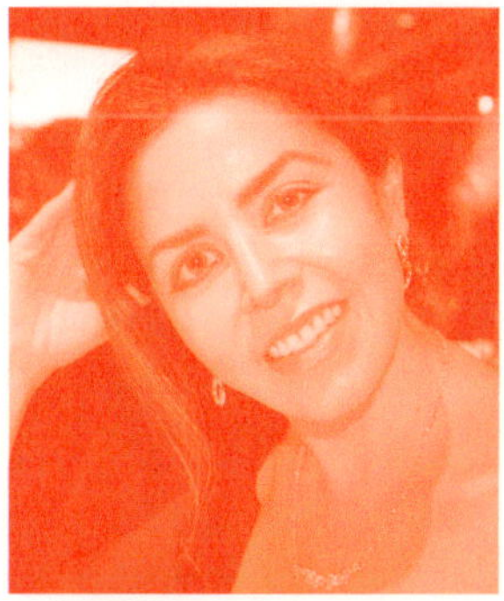

Supporting open minds since 2005

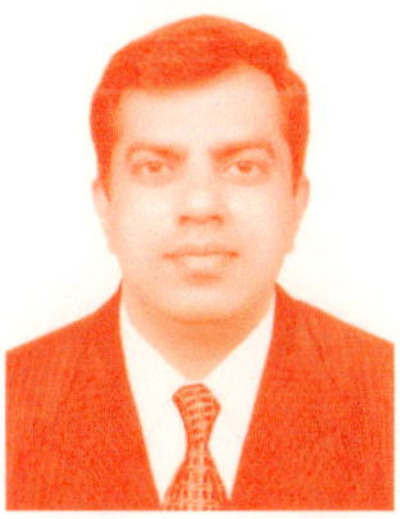
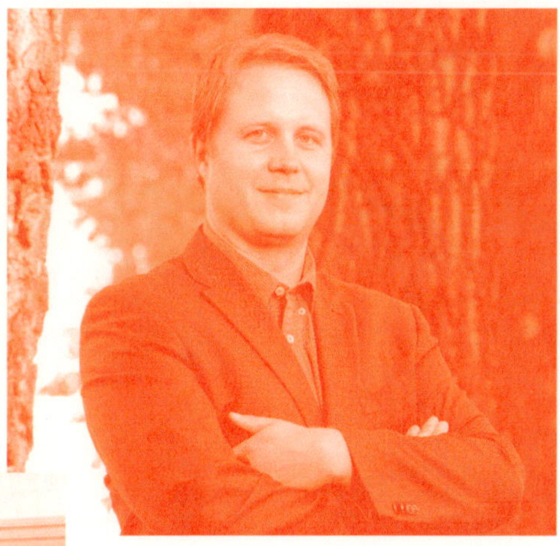
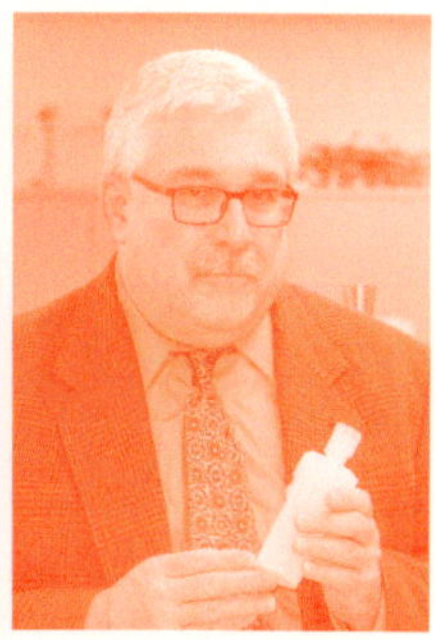
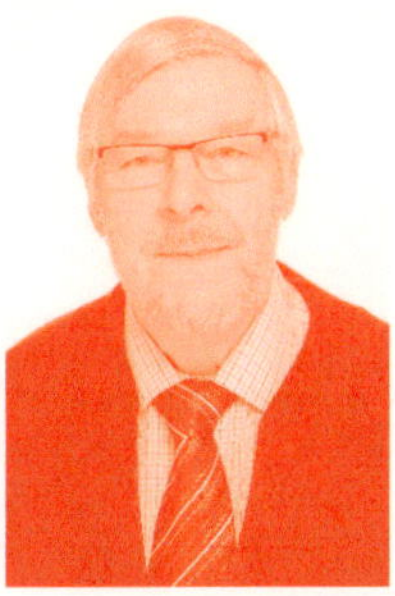
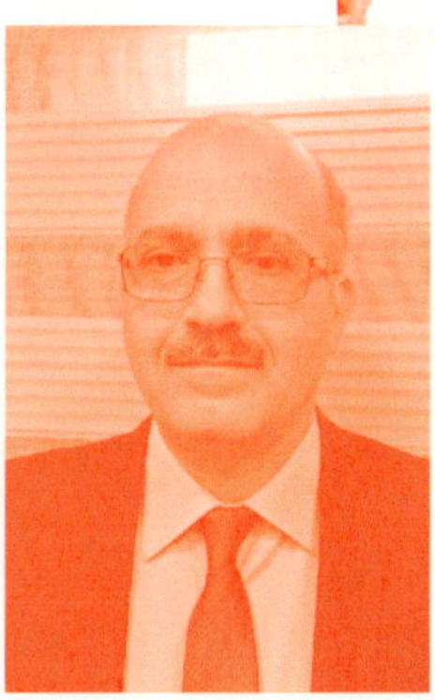
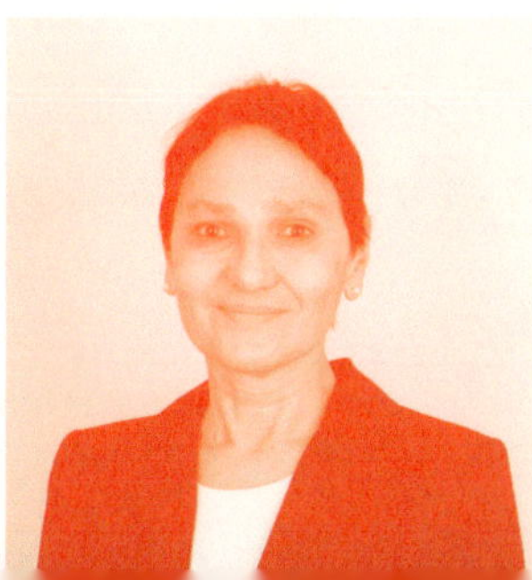
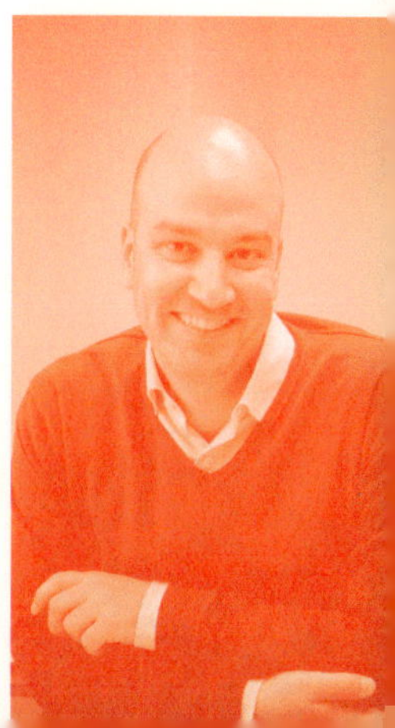

Neurosurgical Procedures - Innovative Approaches
http://dx.doi.org/10.5772/intechopen.78468
Edited by Alba Scerrati and Pasquale De Bonis

Contributors
Michael E. Ivan, Ashish Shah, Daniel Eichberg, Evan Luther, Michael Kader, Alexa Semonche, Katherine Berry, Long Di, Asifur Rahman, Mayank Kaushal, Hoon Choi, Shekar Kurpad, Giuseppe Maria Della Pepa, Alba Scerrati, Oriela Rustemi, Alessandro Della Puppa, Frank Y. Shan, Wan-Ming Hu, Sanjib Mukherjee, Danijela Levacic, Jason H. Huang

First published in London, United Kingdom, 2020 by IntechOpen
IntechOpen is the global imprint of INTECHOPEN LIMITED, registered in England and Wales, registration number: 11086078, 7th floor, 10 Lower Thames Street, London, EC3R 6AF, United Kingdom
Printed in Croatia

British Library Cataloguing-in-Publication Data
A catalogue record for this book is available from the British Library

Additional hard and PDF copies can be obtained from orders@intechopen.com

Neurosurgical Procedures - Innovative Approaches
Edited by Alba Scerrati and Pasquale De Bonis
p. cm.
Print ISBN 978-1-78985-927-0
Online ISBN 978-1-78985-928-7
eBook (PDF) ISBN 978-1-78985-111-3

For EU product safety concerns:
IN TECH d.o.o., Prolaz Marije Krucifikse Kozulić 3, 51000 Rijeka, Croatia, info@intechopen.com or visit our website at intechopen.com.

Meet the editors

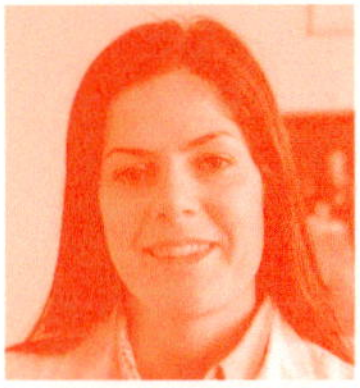

Dr. Alba Scerrati was born in Rome, where she lived until 2017. She then moved to Ferrara. She graduated from medical school in 2010 and completed her neurosurgical residency (in 2017) in the Catholic University of Rome, Policlinico Gemelli. She is Assistant Professor of Neurosurgery at the University of Ferrara where she also works as a neurosurgeon. Dr. Scerrati's main scientific interests are in skull base surgery and neurovascular surgery. She is currently working on the development of 3D printing techniques for neurovascular surgery training and simulation. She is the author and co-author of more than 30 indexed publications (https://www.ncbi.nlm.nih.gov/pubmed/?term=scerrati+a).

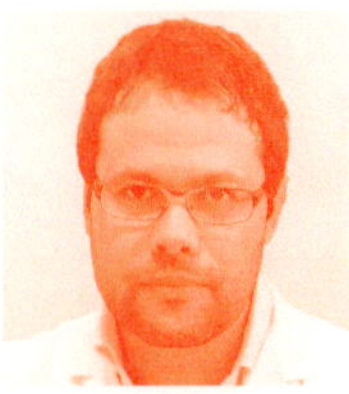

Prof. Pasquale De Bonis has been Associate Professor of Neurosurgery at the University of Ferrara and Head of the Neurosurgery Residency Program since 2017. He graduated cum laude in 2004 from the Medical School at the Catholic University of Rome, Policlinico Gemelli. He completed his residency in neurosurgery in 2009 and his PhD in Neurosciences in 2012 at the Catholic University of Rome. Prof. De Bonis's main scientific interests are in neuroncology, CSF dynamics, and spinal diseases. He is the author and co-author of more than 150 indexed publications (https://www.ncbi.nlm.nih.gov/pubmed/?term=de+bonis+p).

Contents

Preface

“There are no constraints on the human mind, no walls around the human spirit, no barriers to our progress except those we ourselves erect.” (Ronald Reagan)

The history of neurosurgery is characterized by a strong relationship with technology. From the introduction of the operating microscope to the development of endoscopes or exoscopes; from the CT scan to the new 3T MRI; from standard ultrasounds to modern high-definition navigated ultrasounds; from intraoperative DSA to new indocyanine video-angiography; and from custom bone reconstruction to 3D printed skull protheses.

Surgery needs technologies to improve its results and the clinical outcome of patients. New generations of surgeons should be trained in the use of new technologies and be open minded towards what tools biomedical engineering or basic science could offer to improve surgical practice.

This book is designed to be a comprehensive introduction to new developments and techniques in neurosurgery and to their application in clinical practice.

Appreciation is due to Prof. Pasquale De Bonis for helping me in this enjoyable task, to Dr. Flavia Dones for her unfailing support and wise counsel, and to Prof. Michele A. Cavallo for his tireless commitment to making me a better surgeon.

Dr. Alba Scerrati
Department of Morphology, Experimental Medicine and Surgery,
Department of Neurosurgery,
University of Ferrara,
Italy

Pasquale De Bonis
Professor,
University of Ferrara,
Italy

Section 1

Surgery

Chapter 1

Robotic-Assisted Systems for Spinal Surgery

Mayank Kaushal, Shekar Kurpad and Hoon Choi

Abstract

Robotic-assisted spinal surgery is in its infancy. It aims to improve the accuracy of screw placement, lower the risk of surgical complications, and reduce radiation exposure to the patient and the surgical team. The present chapter attempts to provide an overview of the evolution of robotic-assisted spinal surgery and highlights different commercially available spine robotic systems in present use. The review concludes with future applications of robotics in spinal surgery.

Keywords: robotics, spine surgery, pedicle screws, radiation, shared-control system, CT scans, fluoroscopy

1. Introduction

Stereotaxy was coined by Victor Horsley and Robert Clarke in 1908 to describe a method of locating points within the brain by using the Cartesian coordinate system that measures distance from a fixed reference point derived from external cranial landmarks [1]. This was followed by the development of image guidance in 1986, which integrated stereotaxy with computed tomography [2]. The development happened in the backdrop of transition from frame-based to frameless stereotaxy based on enhancements in spatial fidelity of imaging data, computational power, and 3-D digitizers [3]. However, spinal surgery applications of the image guidance systems arising from these refinements carry limitations. These include dependence on a direct line of sight between the optical tracking system and navigated instruments for ensuring screw insertion accuracy and a learning curve for using the navigation system. The learning curve comes from the fact that the surgeon now has to redirect his or her eyes from the patient to the navigation screen in order to follow the planned trajectory for screw placement. This can result in surgical errors since attention is taken away from the patient at the point of screw insertion. An attempt to address this shortcoming has led to the development of robotic systems that utilize similar image guidance platforms while physically guiding the surgeon to the preplanned trajectory for screw placement [4, 5].

The field of spinal surgery is characterized by a unique set of defining features such as the need for high order of surgical precision as several critical structures are located in close proximity of the vertebral column. Injury to these structures, which include blood vessels and nerves, can lead to a wide spectrum of consequences ranging from pain to paralysis. The close association of critical structures is compounded by the narrow operating corridors for doing surgeries involving the spinal column. This set of challenging circumstances strengthens the case for robots as surgical assistants due to the lack of fatigability while undertaking tasks repeatedly and without showing a reduction in performance. Since the introduction of da Vinci Surgical System (Intuitive Surgical, Sunnyvale, CA), cleared for use by the Food and Drug Administration (FDA) in 2000, the field of robotic surgery has continued to mature and gain more widespread acceptance. However, the field of neurosurgery has seen growing interest only in recent times for the use of surgical robotic systems to assist the surgeon in operative procedures.

With surgical robots becoming more visible in a number of surgical disciplines, the various systems in use can be broadly classified into three main categories depending on the interaction of the surgeon with the robot [3]. The first category is supervisory-controlled systems where the actions carried out by the robot are preprogrammed by the surgeon who then monitors the robot performing the specified steps autonomously. The second type is the telesurgical systems where the surgical manipulator follows the movements of an input device directly manipulated by the surgeon in a master-slave manner. The third type is the shared-control models where the motions are concurrently controlled by both the surgeon and the robot via shared control of the surgical instruments. Despite the shared control, the surgeon remains in charge of the decision-making related to the procedure with the robot providing steady-hand manipulation of the instruments [3]. All the surgical robots approved by the FDA for spinal procedures fall under the third category of shared-control systems.

To this point, robotics have largely been utilized in placement of pedicle screws and shown comparable and/or superior accuracy of screw placement compared to conventional, freehand technique of screw placement [6–8]. Despite the initial encouraging findings, the adoption of surgical robots has been relatively slow among the spine surgical community with robots not yet considered as part of the routine standard operative procedure for spinal indications. A major concern for the tepid response to robots is the significant capital investments required for the surgical robot and the associated navigation equipment. The use of navigation systems irrespective of surgical robots is still not commonplace across the surgical suites, which places training requirements on top of the added cost. Further compounding the situation is the perception that adding steps to the operation workflow would lead to increased operation time and decreased efficiency. Given the limited scientific literature on operative and clinical outcomes, there is skepticism toward robots by the surgical community. In the present article, we attempt to explore the evolution of robotic-assisted spinal surgery to where the field stands now and conclude with future applications.

2. Commercial surgical robotic systems in current use

The last two decades have seen the introduction of several robotic systems in spinal surgery but the Food and Drug Administration approval has been granted to three of these systems (**Figure 1**). These include SpineAssist® (Medtronic Inc., Dublin, Ireland), ROSA® (Medtech S.A., Montpellier, France), and ExcelsiusGPS® (Globus Medical Inc., Audubon, PA). SpineAssist®, which received both FDA clearance and European CE Mark of approval in 2004, was the first robotic assistance system to be used in the spinal surgery. Subsequent iterations of SpineAssist®, Renaissance®, and Mazor X™ were released to address some of the limitations of SpineAssist® and received both FDA and CE approval in 2011 and 2017, respectively. The most recent follow-up of SpineAssist® is Mazor X™ Stealth Edition, which received FDA clearance in 2018. The second system approved for commercial use, ROSA®, obtained CE Mark of approval in 2014 FDA clearance in 2016, while the most recent surgical robot system, ExcelsiusGPS®, received both FDA and CE approvals in 2017.

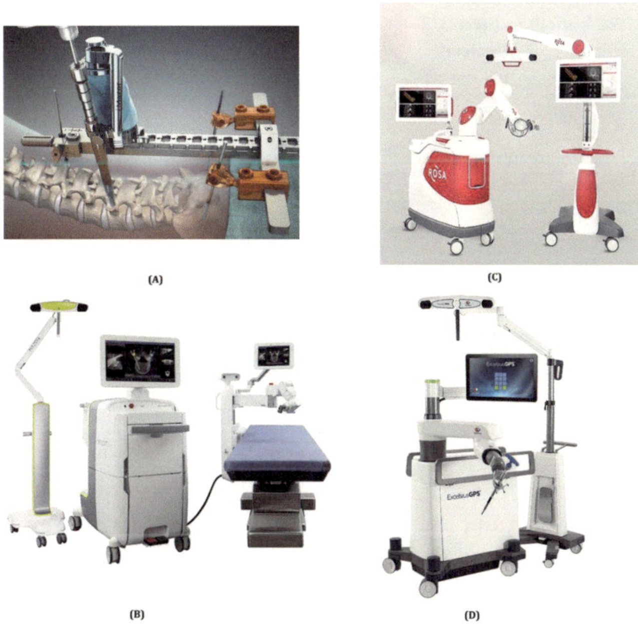

Figure 1.
Systems for robotic-assisted spine surgery: Mazor Renaissance® (A), Mazor X™ (B), ROSA® (C), and ExcelsiusGPS® (D).

2.1 SpineAssist®

SpineAssist® was the first commercially available system for robotic-assisted spinal surgery. It comprises a cylindrical device mounted to a patient-specific anatomical landmark, which relies on pre- and/or intraoperative CT imaging to allow trajectory planning for screw insertion. Subsequent iterations of SpineAssist® include Renaissance® followed by Mazor X™ (list price ~US$1.2 M) with the latter consisting of an independent robotic arm where the attachment to the patient is done using a single pin in place of a robot-mounted platform as is the case with the former. Medtronic Stealth System is used concurrently to provide navigation. Recently, Mazor X™ Stealth Edition has been released, which also obviates the need for K-wires and a separate navigation system. Like the previous versions, it requires the robotic arm to be mounted to the bedframe.

2.2 ROSA®

The second system approved by the FDA is the ROSA®, which works similar to the SpineAssist® in using pre- or intraoperative CT imaging to plan screw trajectory but provides the additional convenience of built-in navigation for determination of screw depth.

2.3 ExcelsiusGPS®

ExcelsiusGPS®, the third and most recently approved commercial robotic system (list price ~US$1.2 M), has a built-in navigation system similar to ROSA® but does not require attachment to the patient or the operating table. In addition, it removes the need for a K-wire by providing an end effector for the passage of instruments and detecting "skiving" of instruments. There is also a secondary passive reflective marker to monitor the accuracy of robotic navigation system.

Robotic system	Navigation	Direct implant placement	K-wire required	Imaging			Portability
				Intra-op	Pre-op	Fluoroscopy	
Renaissance	Separate	No	Yes		✓		Patient mounted
Mazor X	Separate	No	Yes	✓	✓		Bed mounted
Mazor X Stealth Edition	Integrated	Yes	No	✓	✓		Bed mounted
ROSA	Integrated	No	Yes	✓			Free standing
ExcelsiusGPS	Integrated	Yes	No	✓	✓	✓	Free standing

Table 1.
Comparison of commercially available spine robotic systems.

Table 1 highlights salient features of each of the surgical robotic systems.

In the subsequent section, the experience with the use of these systems is described followed by an appraisal of the limitations of the present systems and avenues for future research. Due to relative longevity of SpineAssist® availability for commercial application, a significant portion of the published literature is based on the experience of using SpineAssist® and its subsequent iterations, Renaissance® and Mazor X™.

3. Applications of robotics in spinal surgery

3.1 Pedicle screw instrumentation

Despite being the most commonly performed procedure related to the thoracolumbar spine, a steep learning curve is associated with transpedicular fixation. Subsequently, the primary application of surgical robots in spinal surgery has been transpedicular fixation. The use of robotic surgical assistants in transpedicular fixation arose from the wide variability of findings about accuracy of screw placements reported for various versions of conventional, fluoroscopic-dependent techniques. The results on the accuracy of pedicle screw instrumentation using surgical robotic assistants have been largely superior to the manual screw insertion using fluoroscopy. The commonly accepted method of determining insertion accuracy involves the use of postoperative CT scans, which despite providing radiographic confirmation of screw placement is limited in divulging the clinical implications of the radiographic findings. This limits the inferences that can be drawn to some extent, but given the popularity of this method of comparison, the various robotic systems are discussed with respect to screw insertion accuracy.

A detailed evaluation of the scientific literature highlights that a significant share of studies document results from SpineAssist® and its iterations, namely, Renaissance® and Mazor X™. The first account on the use of robotics was provided by Sukovich et al. in a 2006 retrospective analysis, which used SpineAssist® in 14 patients for the placement of 98 pedicle screws through a combination of open and minimally invasive techniques. The authors showed that 96% of the screws were within 1–2 mm of the planned trajectory with no cases of pedicle breach [9]. In another study, Pechlivanis et al. looked at the screw insertion accuracy of SpineAssist® during minimally invasive posterior lumbar interbody fusion (PLIF). The accuracy was determined on postoperative CT scans using the Gertzbein and Robbins system (GRS) for evaluating the accuracy of pedicle screw insertion [10, 11]. The GRS grades the screws into four categories based on the location of the screw within the pedicle: Grade A, screw is completely within the pedicle; Grade B, screw breach is <2 mm; Grade C, screw breach is >2 and <4 mm; Grade D, screw breach is >4 and <6 mm; and Grade E, screw breach is >6 mm. Grades A and B are considered acceptable for screw accuracy. Of the 122 screws inserted, with the exception of one screw that was Grade D, the remaining screws were either GRS Grade A (108) or GRS Grade B [13]. Devito et al. performed a multicenter, retrospective review comprising of 3271 pedicle screws placed with SpineAssist® and showed 98% of the screw insertions to be acceptable when assessed by intraoperative fluoroscopy. Further, accuracy measurements done on postoperative CT scans in a subset of these screws (646) showed over 98% of the screws fell within the safe zone (GRS Grades A and B) [12]. In a study involving 112 patients and 494 screws using SpineAssist®, van Dijk and colleagues found a 97.9% rate of clinically acceptable screw insertion [13]. Hu et al. evaluated 960 pedicle screws placed with Renaissance® and found that 949 screws (98.9%) were placed accurately [14]. A separate study by the same group showed successful screw placement in nine patients with spinal column tumors [15]. In a review of 50 patients with adolescent idiopathic scoliosis (AIS) that underwent robotic MIS posterior spinal fusion, Macke et al. evaluated a total of 662 pedicle screws inserted using Renaissance®. The authors observed a 92.7% acceptable placement rate. Lower rates of screw malpositioning were noted with robotic MIS than prior published data, and improved accuracy of screw insertion was observed when using preoperative CT obtained in the prone position [16].

A number of studies have compared accuracy between conventional freehand and robotic-assisted procedures. In a retrospective analysis, Kantelhardt et al. used SpineAssist® and performed pedicle screw placement accuracy comparisons between three groups, namely, conventional freehand versus open robotic-assisted versus percutaneous robotic-assisted, and showed comparable accuracy rates for the combined robotic-assisted groups (94.5%) and the freehand group (91.4%) for screw insertion [17]. Schatlo and colleagues used SpineAssist® and demonstrated similar rates of clinically acceptable screw placement between open fluoroscopy-guided and robotic-assisted placement (open and percutaneous) groups [18]. In a separate analysis by the same group, the impact of experience of surgeon on screw insertion accuracy was evaluated for 1265 pedicle screws. The authors showed 1217 (96.2%) screw placements were of an acceptable grade with screw misplacement peaking between the first 10 and 20 surgeries and declining as more surgeries were performed by the surgeon [19]. The same group followed this up with an analysis involving 169 patients that underwent posterior instrumentation for spinal instability and showed a higher proportion of non-misplaced screws in the robot (93.4%) than the freehand fluoroscopy-guided cohort (88.9%), which was statistically significant [20]. Schizas et al. evaluated robot-assisted (open or percutaneous) versus fluoroscopy cohort and showed comparable accuracy rates with 95.3% for the robotics group and 92.2% for the freehand group [21]. The accuracy of screw insertion was assessed using the Rampersaud scale, which describes the relative position of the screw to the pedicle and comprises the following four grades: Grade A, completely in; Grade B, <2 mm breach; Grade C, 2–4 mm breach; and Grade D, >4 mm breach [22]. Solomiichuk and colleagues performed a retrospective matched cohort study in 70 patients diagnosed with metastatic spine disease and showed grade A or B screw placement in 162 of 192 (84.4%) in the robotic-assisted group and in 179 of 214 (83.6%) in the conventional group with no differences in screw accuracy between the groups. Further, no differences were found between the cohorts for accuracy, duration of surgery, radiation exposure, or surgical site infection with the exception of intensity of radiation [23]. Keric et al. evaluated 90 patients treated for spondylodiscitis with posterior spinal fusion via either conventional, open freehand, or percutaneous robot-assisted spinal instrumentation using Renaissance®. Their findings revealed robotic cohort was associated with higher accuracy and lower likelihood for revision procedures for improper screw placement. Further, the robotic-assisted MIS cohort had lower intraoperative fluoroscopy and shorter postoperative stay [24]. In a separate review of 1857 implanted screws, Keric and colleagues showed increased rates of screw deviation in clinical diagnosis such as tumor, infection, and osteoporotic fractures [25]. In another review of 206 patients with spondylodiscitis that underwent posterior spinal fusion, Alaid et al. observed a lower rate of revision for wound breakdown in the robotic MIS group using SpineAssist® than the open, freehand group [26].

The comparison of screw accuracy between freehand and robotic-guided screw insertion has also been analyzed through a number of randomized controlled trials. Kim et al. compared the accuracy and safety of screw insertion between robotic-assisted minimally invasive PLIF using Renaissance® (37 patients) and conventional, freehand technique for PLIF (41 patients). For intrapedicular accuracy, no significant differences were observed between the groups. Of the 74 screws in the robotic cohort, none breached the proximal facet joint, while 13 of the 82 screws in the freehand group violated the proximal facet joint ($P < 0.001$). Further, the average distance of the screws from the left and right facets was significantly smaller in the freehand group [27]. Roser et al. used SpineAssist® to compare screw accuracy between fluoroscopic-guided freehand, navigation-guided, and robotic-assisted screw instrumentation. The authors found no significant differences for screw accuracy between the different techniques, but the conclusion was not backed by statistical analysis due to small study size [28]. Ringel et al. compared an equal number of patients randomly assigned to either percutaneous screw placement using SpineAssist® or conventional, open freehand technique. The results of their RCT differ from the large majority of studies in that a lower rate (85%) of clinically acceptable screw placement was reported for robotic-guided technique than the freehand technique (93%) for screw insertion [29]. Hyun and colleagues performed a prospective study comparing fluoroscopy-guided approach with MIS screw insertion using Renaissance® in lumbar fusions. The authors observed all screws in the robotic group were placed accurately, while in the freehand group, the accuracy rate was 98.6% [30]. In a prospective analysis, Park and colleagues compared 37 patients with MIS screw insertion using Renaissance® and 41 patients that underwent freehand technique for pedicle screw insertion during posterior interbody fusion surgery. They showed both groups had similar improvement in clinical outcomes at 2-year follow-up [31].

Aside from studies on SpineAssist® and its iterations, only a small number of publications have explored other surgical systems. Lonjon et al. compared screw placement using the ROSA® with freehand technique of screw insertion. The authors found a 97.2% accuracy rate in the robotic group and a 92% accuracy rate in the freehand group [32]. In a study by Huntsman et al., MIS screw placement using ExcelsiusGPS® showed 99% of screw placed successfully based on the surgeon's interpretation of intraoperative plain film radiographs, with no cases of screw malposition requiring revision surgery [33].

3.2 Other applications

Bederman et al. evaluated the utility of SpineAssist® or Renaissance® robotic system in the placement of S2-alar-iliac screws and found all screws are placed accurately with no breach of the anterior sacrum [34]. Hu et al. performed a retrospective analysis of 18 patients who underwent S2AI fixation with assistance from Renaissance® robotic system and found accurate screw trajectory on postoperative CT scans without any violations of iliac cortex or breaches of the anterior sacrum [35]. In another study comprising of four adult spinal deformity patients who underwent minimally invasive robotic-guided insertion of S2-alar-iliac (S2AI) screws using Renaissance® robotic system, Hyun et al. observed all the screw trajectories were positioned accurately based on postoperative X-rays and CT scans [36]. Laratta and colleagues evaluated S2AI screw insertion in 23 consecutive patients who underwent spinopelvic fixation with Renaissance® robotic system and noted two violations of iliac cortex but no neurologic, vascular, or visceral complications among the 46 S2AI screws that were inserted [37]. In a retrospective matched cohort analysis, Shillingford et al. compared robotic-assisted using Renaissance® robotic system (23 patients, 46 screws) and conventional, freehand (28 patients, 59 screws) S2AI screw placement in 68 consecutive patients with spinal deformity. The authors observed no differences between the groups for screw insertion accuracy or intraoperative complications [38].

4. Illustrative case examples

4.1 Case 1: MIS robotic-assisted thoracolumbar instrumentation for adult trauma

A 44-year-old healthy man presented to the hospital following a 12-ft fall from the roof of a house while repairing it. He complained of severe back pain with right-sided leg numbness. Physical examination demonstrated severe pain and numbness in the lower limbs. On CT, a burst fracture at L1 was observed with MRI showing injury to the posterior ligamentous complex (PLC) (**Figure 2**). The decision-making for the clinical management for the patient was evaluated using the thoracolumbar injury classification and severity score (TLICS), a classification system for thoracolumbar injuries that predicts the need for surgery [39]. It comprises three independent predictors, which are morphology, integrity of PLC, and neurological status. The patient presentation was given a TLICS score of 7, and consequently the patient underwent robotic-assisted MIS T11-L3 fixation and fusion (**Figure 3**). The patient had complete recovery.

4.2 Case 2: open robotic-assisted thoracolumbar fusion for pediatric trauma

A 13-year-old boy presented to the hospital after landing on his upper back while attempting to jump out of a swinging hammock. He reported thoracolumbar pain, which was located in the hip region but had no radicular pain into the lower abdomen

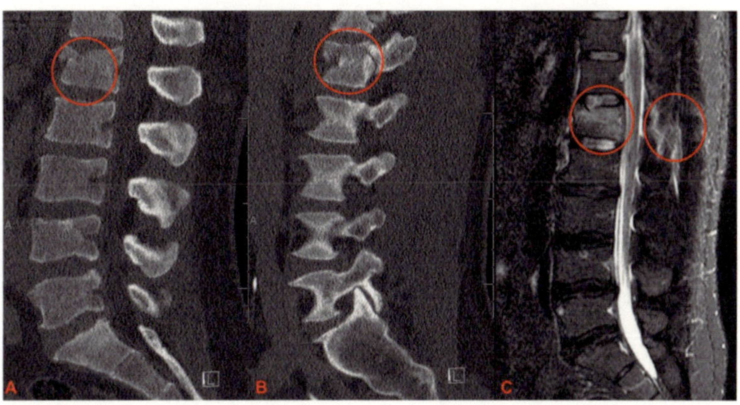

Figure 2.
Case 1: Preoperative CT (A and B) and MRI (C) showing L1 burst fracture with injury to the posterior ligamentous complex (red circles).

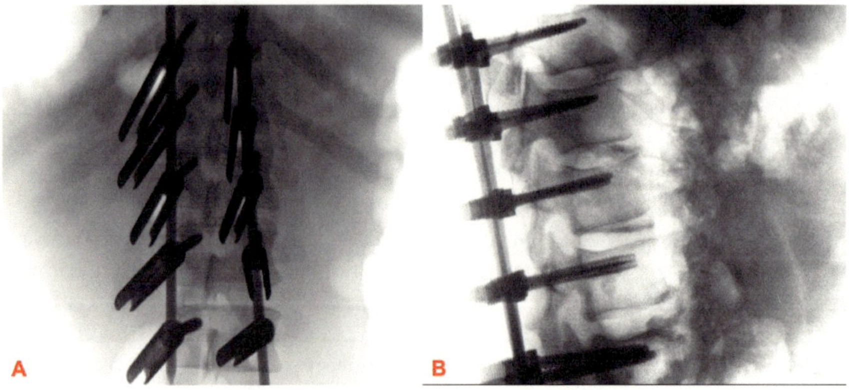

Figure 3.
Case 1: Intraoperative X-rays showing MIS T11–L3 transpedicular fixation (A and B).

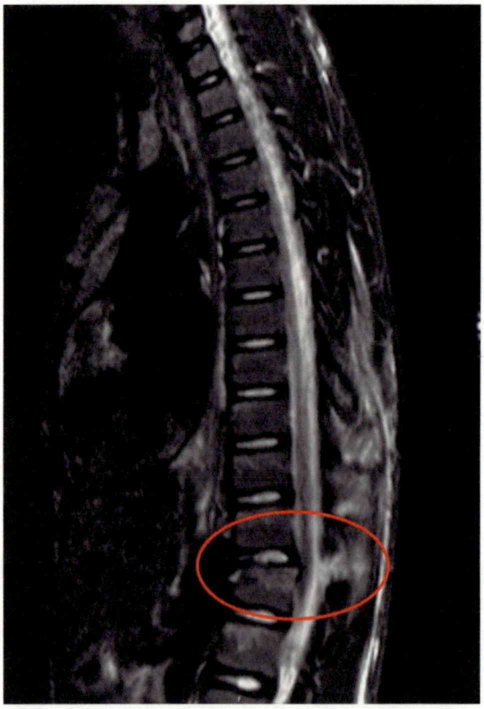

Figure 4.
Case 2: Preoperative MRI showing T11–T12 anterolisthesis, T12 wedge fracture with T11–T12 facet dislocation, and posterior ligamentous injury with small dorsal epidural hematoma (red circle).

or legs. MRI revealed T11/T12 anterolisthesis, T12 wedge fracture with T11–T12 facet dislocation, and posterior ligamentous injury with small dorsal epidural hematoma (**Figure 4**). CT thoracic spine showed fracture and subluxation at T11–T12 with bilateral perched T11 facets, right pedicle fracture of T12 extending into the superior end plate of the vertebral body with wedging of T12 along with anterior and inferior displacement of the anterior ring apophysis, and spinous process fractures of T11 and to a lesser extent T10 (**Figure 5**). Based on the clinical presentation and imaging findings, a decision to operate was made. The patient underwent robotic-assisted T10-L1 fixation and fusion, T11/T12 open reduction and internal fixation at T11–T12, and T11 laminotomy for epidural hematoma evacuation (**Figure 6**). The patient had complete recovery and subsequently underwent removal of the hardware at 1 year.

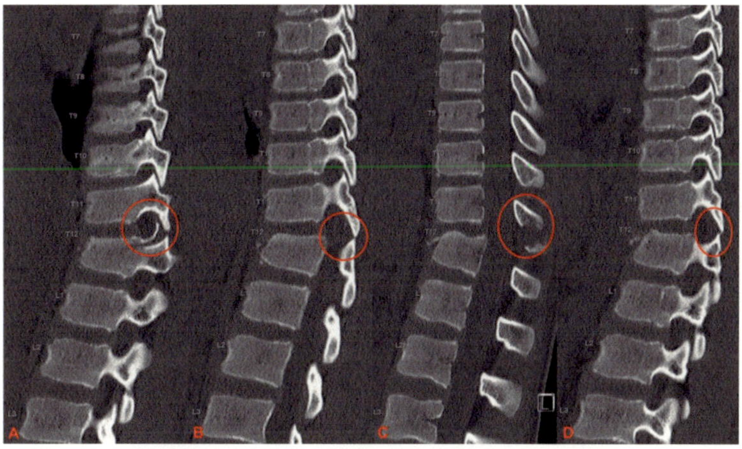

Figure 5.
Case 2: Preoperative CT thoracic spine (A–D) showing bilateral T11–T12 facet dislocation, bilateral perched facets, and T10 spinous process fracture (red circles).

4.3 Case 3: MIS robotic-assisted TLIF for degenerative spine

A 58-year-old female presented to the hospital with back and leg pain. The leg pain was on the left side and radiating to the left foot. The patient mentioned the back pain was worse than the left lower extremity (LLE) pain with duration of pain progressing over the last 2 years. Additionally, she complained of LLE weakness and numbness as well as cramping in bilateral calf muscles. Imaging showed 11 mm L4/5 anterolisthesis on standing XR (**Figure 7**) and severe spinal stenosis at L4/5 on MRI (**Figure 8**). Her medication history included hydrocodone, meloxicam, and tizanidine. Due to the long duration of the pain, the patient had tried a number of conservative treatments such as chiropractic, transcutaneous electrical nerve stimulation (TENS), and heat/ice packs but mentioned that none of these treatments had

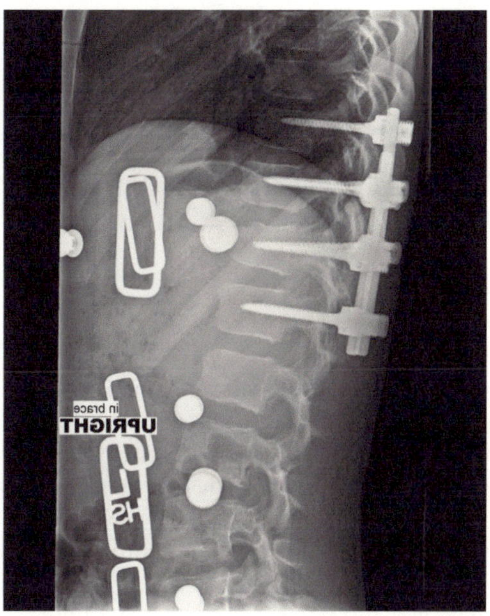

Figure 6.
Case 2: Postoperative X-ray showing T10–L1 transpedicular fixation and restoration of spinal alignment.

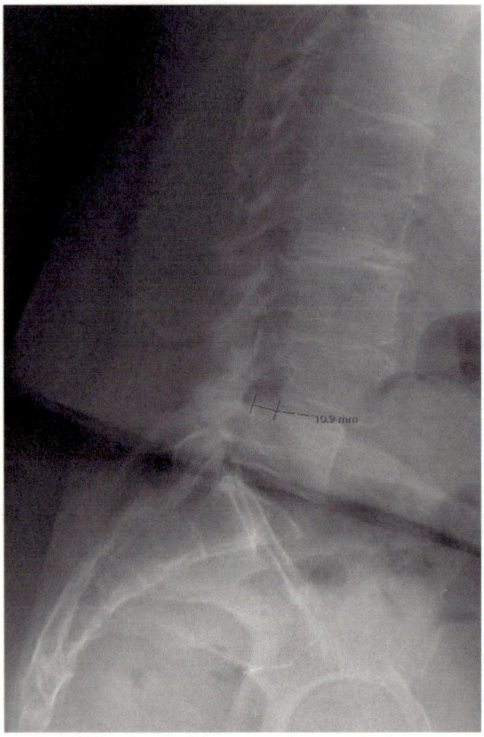

Figure 7.
Case 3: Preoperative standing X-ray showing 11 mm L4/5 anterolisthesis.

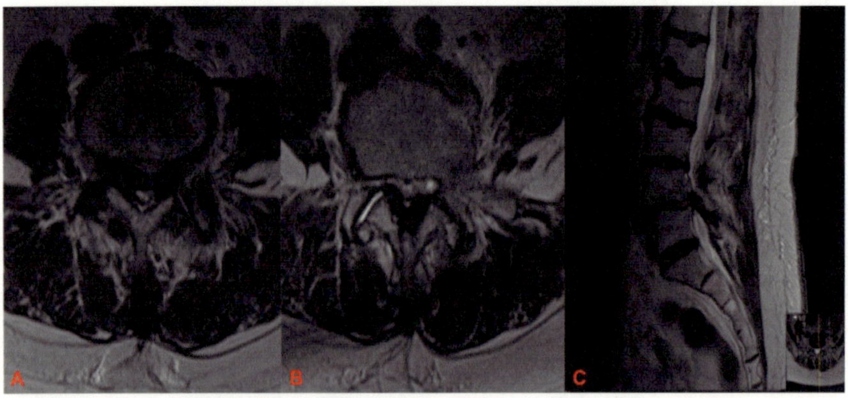

Figure 8.
Case 3: Preoperative MRI in axial (A and B) and sagittal (C) planes showing severe spinal canal, lateral recess, and foraminal stenoses at L4–5.

worked for her. Based on the clinical presentation and imaging findings, a decision to surgical operation was made, and the patient underwent an MIS robotic-assisted transforaminal lumbar interbody fusion (TLIF, **Figure 9**). The patient was discharged within a day and had resolution of back and leg symptoms on follow-up.

4.4 Case 4: hybrid MIS robotic-assisted cervicothoracic fusion for adult trauma

A 30-year-old female presented to the hospital after being involved in a rollover motor vehicle accident. Physical examination demonstrated severe neck pain and tingling in the left arm. On imaging, she had left C5–C6 facet fracture dislocation

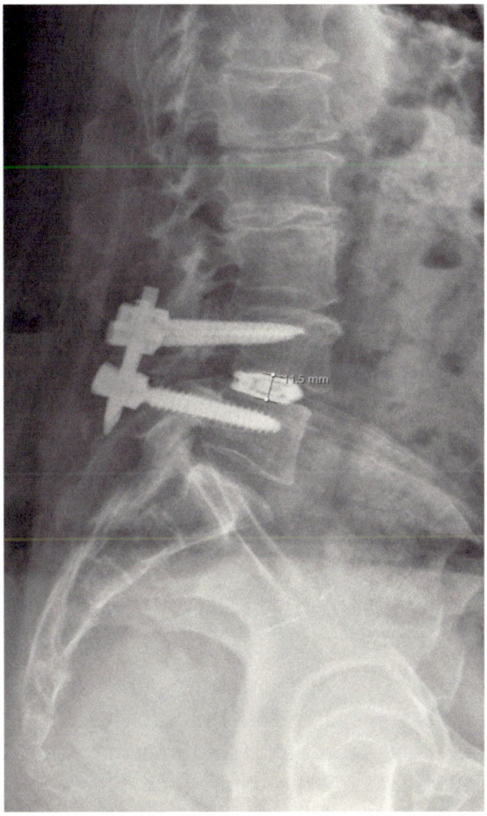

Figure 9.
Case 3: Postoperative standing X-ray showing L4–5 transforaminal lumbar interbody fusion with spondylolisthesis reduction and disc height restoration.

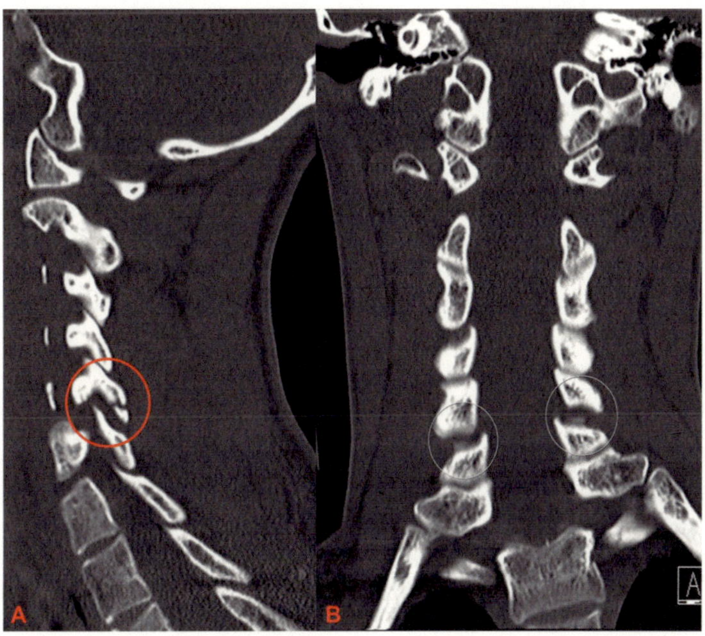

Figure 10.
Case 4: Preoperative CT showing C5–C6 facet fracture dislocation and bilateral C5–C6 facet distraction (red and gray circles).

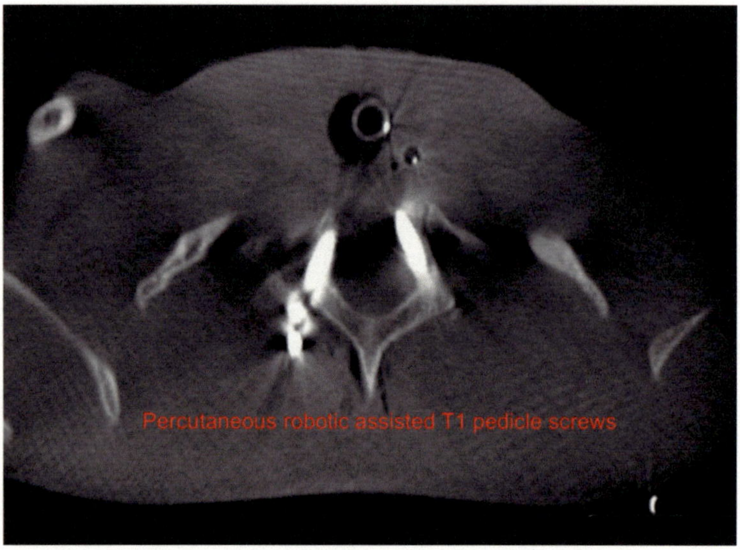

Figure 11.
Case 4: Intraoperative CT showing percutaneous robotic-assisted T1 pedicle screws.

and bilateral C5–C6 facet distraction (**Figure 10**). The patient underwent C4-T1 fixation and fusion with percutaneous MIS robotic-assisted T1 pedicle screws (**Figure 11**). Her midline incision could be minimized to approximately 3 inches. She had complete recovery and was discharged to the rehabilitation unit.

5. Discussion and future directions

Radiation exposure is an important consideration when comparing the utility of robotics in spinal surgery to conventional, fluoroscopic techniques. With expanding indications for the use of MIS in more complex spinal cases, the concern about radiation is a major factor in technology adoption going forward. Recognizing the impact of this issue on increased adoption of robotics, a number of studies have looked at the radiation exposure in patients operated with the assistance from surgical robotics vis-à-vis patients treated with conventional, fluoroscopic techniques. Based on the limited literature on this topic, it appears the incorporation of robots in the operating workflow is associated with reduction in both the time and the levels of radiation exposure [40]. In a prospective randomized controlled trial, Hyun et al. observed shorter radiation times and output in the robotic group, which was statistically significant [30]. Kim and colleagues noted a significant reduction in fluoroscopy duration in later cases when compared to the early cases [41]. In a study comparing different guiding methods for pedicle screw insertion, Fan et al. showed that robotic-assisted technique was associated with shorter fluoroscopic time than conventional, freehand technique or O-arm-based navigation but longer time than patient-specific navigational template technique [42]. Another study looking at different screw insertion guiding techniques showed the lowest dose of radiation in the standard navigation group, which was followed by the robotic group and then the conventional, freehand group [28]. Kantelhardt et al. found that robotic-assisted screw insertion had statistically significant lower radiation exposure than conventional, freehand technique. However, the authors found no difference between percutaneous and open robotic-assisted pedicle screw insertion [17]. Similarly, Keric and colleagues noted lower fluoroscopy time in the robotic-assisted screw insertion cohort [24]. In contrast, Ringel et al. and Schizas et al. found no differences in radiation exposure between the robotic and the freehand groups [21, 29]. Based on published data, it appears that robotic-assisted procedures lead to reduction in radiation exposure with the greatest value addition of robots being in percutaneous screw insertion. The use of robots in this case has the potential to reduce the radiation exposure, which tends to increase dramatically for conventional screw insertion techniques. The end result of incorporating robotics could obviate the need for lead apron by the operating room staff.

When compared with navigation, the use of robotics allows for preplanning of screws. This saves operative time and allows the operating room staff to prepare implants ahead of time. By preparing for any anatomical variations that the surgeon might encounter (such as in deformity, trauma, and previously arthrodesed spines), the robot can be deployed for spinal procedures that involve more complex anatomical relationships. Over time, enhancements to graphical user interface have simplified the screw trajectory planning. By allowing the superimposition of intraoperative scans over preoperative imaging, the robots help the surgeon to take into consideration patient movement to more accurately plan the procedure while also providing the surgeon with the ability to select optimal screw dimensions. By taking into account patient immobilization, a robotic surgical assistant can lead to a diminished operating time while reducing pedicle and vertebral body violations. Further, the visualization provided by the robotic software platform can aid in rod contouring/placement through optimized screw cadence and skin incision optimization for MIS procedures in obese patients.

The experience with the use of surgical robots in spine surgery has been positive so far with a large majority of studies documenting outcomes observed with robots that are equal or superior to the findings observed with conventional, openhand technique. This is on account of the reduction of human manual error as the robot provides a stable, rigid channel for guiding surgical instruments by the surgeon. The same advantage holds true when compared to navigation-assisted screw placement, which is more prone to deviations due to lack of a stable conduit for maneuvering instruments. Further, the ability to lock trajectories allows for repeatability during surgical procedures by limiting the influence of physiological hand tremor, which allows for efficiency gains over time. This element of repeatability has the added benefit of providing the surgeon the ability to better plan skin incisions. Despite the possible advantages of robots, the capabilities of the present robotic systems are fairly limited, which only favors their role in a narrow, specific set of indications as evident from most of the present literature being on the use of robots for primarily pedicle screw fixation. However, it is crucial to acknowledge the results by Ringel et al. that noted lower screw insertion accuracy with the use of surgical robotic system. A number of possible reasons could have led to these findings including lateral skidding of the cannula at the entrance point caused by the steep slope of the lateral aspect of the facet joint or using a platform fixed to a cranial spinal process with a K-wire and attached to the operating table by a bed mount, which meant the robot was only attached to the patient via a single K-wire [43].

With robotics continuing to become more visible in the spinal surgery, a discussion of future areas of developments is warranted. A major thrust for moving the field of robotics forward would involve arriving at reproducible definitions of screw trajectory that mitigate the interruptions to the surgical workflow caused by the present manual method of trajectory planning. Knez and colleagues employed nonparametric models of vertebral bodies and pedicles registered to the patient CT while also accounting for spinal curvature to calculate automatic trajectories that showed close agreement with manually defined plans [44, 45]. In a study based on an atlas-based method that incorporated patterns of biomechanically optimal constructs and a surgeon's own planning preferences, Vijayan et al. highlighted a method that is generalizable to other surgical planning applications [46]. The abovementioned methods are not only built on the premise of introducing consistency to screw trajectories but also hold potential for the estimation of screw diameter(s) and length(s) to be used in a given operation.

Perhaps the greatest challenge impeding the growth of robotic systems stems from the inability of present systems to utilize visual cues from the surroundings to identify objects both accurately and automatically. Therefore, the functionality of a robot is completely modeled by the humans, and accordingly robots are only able to perform tasks for which they are preconfigured. The present state of affairs shows the path forward, which in all likelihood will see robotics integrating with artificial intelligence (AI) to confer robots with increased accuracy in visual identification and autonomous decision-making capacity. This would entail competing with visual systems seen in humans where two-dimensional inputs from the environment are collected by the human eye and converted into three-dimensional interpreted by the brain. Further, the surgical environment is a dynamic one and responding in such a way an environment would need sequential processing of external stimuli in real time. This is necessary for the robots to transition from mere translators of preprogrammed structured scenarios to dynamic adaptors in the external world. The enhancements to spatial and temporal visual information processing capabilities bring to attention the central role of neural networks in bringing these capabilities online. Modeled on the parallel processing structure of the human brain, an artificial neural network is composed of interconnected processing elements. Neural network learning is driven by the training algorithm autonomously and continually adjusting the connection weights based on exposure to input/output data. By being exposed to the surgeon's screw planning preferences, the robot would over time be able to automatically plan the screws for the surgeon. Further, machine learning could be utilized to pool data from several surgeons and make use of their combined expertise to suggest optimized screw trajectories over the cloud, irrespective of the geographical location of the surgeon.

As technological adoption increases among the younger generations of surgeons, virtual reality (VR) platforms for skills acquisition and operative planning among other function would grow in demand. While a virtual depiction of the operating environment is imperative from an educational point of view, the superimposition of virtual objects over real-world environment via hybrid systems known as augmented reality (AR) is needed for enhanced manipulation. An example of such a scenario would perhaps include head-mounted visor that projects screw trajectory in front of the surgeon on a virtual display with the surgeon not located in the immediate vicinity of the patient. This would demand capabilities for seamless, real-time transmission and integration of stereoscopic images defining the operative field and imaging data defining the patient anatomy. The rise of AR could also be instrumental in ushering remote collaboration between surgeons located at distant geographic locations. This would need improvements in information transmission capabilities to allow for real-time collaboration, an area where fifth generation (5G) network technology might be of assistance. However, these developments speak to a more distant future, and in the more immediate time frame, robotics in spinal surgery might come to resemble the da Vinci Surgical System, a slave master system, where the surgeon sits at a console and controls the robot.

Of note, the enhanced capabilities would need to be designed in a manner that makes the robot a hand dexterity enhancer for the surgeon while still being in full control by the surgeon. As robotic technology becomes more sophisticated, the move toward autonomous robots will raise concerns about the transfer of control from the surgeon to the robot and the growing dependence of the surgeon on the in-built systems of the robot. Further, the possibility for real-time collaboration among physicians for screw planning recommendation as well doing the actual screw placement will raise concerns about patient consent, medical liability, and data confidentiality, among others. These are relevant ethical challenges of our time that demand more research into crucial areas of robotic design related to both software and hardware as well as the medicolegal requirements protecting the patient such as the Health Insurance Portability and Accountability Act (HIPAA).

6. Conclusions

The current state of robotics in spinal surgery is comprised of a limited range of clinical indications related to screw placement. With emerging data showing acceptable rates for screw insertion and radiation exposure, the field of robotics is expected to benefit from further technological developments.

Author details

Mayank Kaushal, Shekar Kurpad and Hoon Choi*
Department of Neurosurgery, Medical College of Wisconsin, Milwaukee, USA

*Address all correspondence to: hchoi@mcw.edu

References

[1] Schurr PH, Merrington WR. The Horsley-Clarke stereotaxic apparatus. The British Journal of Surgery. 1978;**65**(1):33-36

[2] Roberts DW, Strohbehn JW, Hatch JF, Murray W, Kettenberger H. A frameless stereotaxic integration of computerized tomographic imaging and the operating microscope. Journal of Neurosurgery. 1986;**65**(4):545-549

[3] Nathoo N, Cavusoglu MC, Vogelbaum MA, Barnett GH, et al. Neurosurgery. 2005;**56**(3):421-433. Discussion 33

[4] Overley SC, Cho SK, Mehta AI, Arnold PM. Navigation and robotics in spinal surgery: Where are we now? Neurosurgery. 2017;**80**(3S):S86-S99

[5] Theodore N, Arnold PM, Mehta AI. Introduction: The rise of the robots in spinal surgery. Neurosurgical Focus. 2018;**45**(VideoSuppl1):Intro

[6] Gao S, Lv Z, Fang H. Robot-assisted and conventional freehand pedicle screw placement: A systematic review and meta-analysis of randomized controlled trials. European Spine Journal. 2018;**27**(4):921-930

[7] Ghasem A, Sharma A, Greif DN, Alam M, Maaieh MA. The arrival of robotics in spine surgery: A review of the literature. Spine. 2018;**43**(23):1670-1677

[8] Fan Y, Du JP, Liu JJ, Zhang JN, Qiao HH, Liu SC, et al. Accuracy of pedicle screw placement comparing robot-assisted technology and the free-hand with fluoroscopy-guided method in spine surgery: An updated meta-analysis. Medicine. 2018;**97**(22):e10970

[9] Sukovich W, Brink-Danan S, Hardenbrook M. Miniature robotic guidance for pedicle screw placement in posterior spinal fusion: Early clinical experience with the SpineAssist. International Journal of Medical Robotics and Computer Assisted Surgery. 2006;**2**(2):114-122

[10] Pechlivanis I, Kiriyanthan G, Engelhardt M, Scholz M, Lucke S, arders A, et al. Percutaneous placement of pedicle screws in the lumbar spine using a bone mounted miniature robotic system: First experiences and accuracy of screw placement. Spine. 2009;**34**(4):392-398

[11] Gertzbein SD, Robbins SE. Accuracy of pedicular screw placement in vivo. Spine. 1990;**15**(1):11-14

[12] Devito DP, Kaplan L, Dietl R, Pfeiffer M, Horne D, Silberstein B, et al. Clinical acceptance and accuracy assessment of spinal implants guided with SpineAssist surgical robot: Retrospective study. Spine. 2010;**35**(24):2109-2115

[13] van Dijk JD, van den Ende RP, Stramigioli S, Kochling M, Hoss N. Clinical pedicle screw accuracy and deviation from planning in robot-guided spine surgery: Robot-guided pedicle screw accuracy. Spine. 2015;**40**(17):E986-E991

[14] Hu X, Ohnmeiss DD, Lieberman IH. Robotic-assisted pedicle screw placement: Lessons learned from the first 102 patients. European Spine Journal. 2013;**22**(3):661-666

[15] Hu X, Scharschmidt TJ, Ohnmeiss DD, Lieberman IH. Robotic assisted surgeries for the treatment of spine tumors. International Journal of Spine Surgery. 2015;**9**:1

[16] Macke JJ, Woo R, Varich L. Accuracy of robot-assisted pedicle screw placement for adolescent idiopathic scoliosis in the pediatric population.

Journal of Robotic Surgery. 2016;**10**(2):145-150

[17] Kantelhardt SR, Martinez R, Baerwinkel S, Burger R, Giese A, Rohde V. Perioperative course and accuracy of screw positioning in conventional, open robotic-guided and percutaneous robotic-guided, pedicle screw placement. European Spine Journal. 2011;**20**(6):860-868

[18] Schatlo B, Molliqaj G, Cuvinciuc V, Kotowski M, Schaller K, Tessitore E. Safety and accuracy of robot-assisted versus fluoroscopy-guided pedicle screw insertion for degenerative diseases of the lumbar spine: A matched cohort comparison. Journal of Neurosurgery. Spine. 2014;**20**(6):636-643

[19] Schatlo B, Martinez R, Alaid A, von Eckardstein K, Akhavan-Sigari R, Hahn A, et al. Acta Neurochirurgica. 2015;**157**(10):1819-1823. Discussion 23

[20] Molliqaj G, Schatlo B, Alaid A, Solomiichuk V, Rohde V, Schaller K, et al. Accuracy of robot-guided versus freehand fluoroscopy-assisted pedicle screw insertion in thoracolumbar spinal surgery. Neurosurgical Focus. 2017;**42**(5):E14

[21] Schizas C, Thein E, Kwiatkowski B, Kulik G. Pedicle screw insertion: Robotic assistance versus conventional C-arm fluoroscopy. Acta Orthopaedica Belgica. 2012;**78**(2):240-245

[22] Rampersaud YR, Pik JH, Salonen D, Farooq S. Clinical accuracy of fluoroscopic computer-assisted pedicle screw fixation: A CT analysis. Spine. 2005;**30**(7):E183-E190

[23] Solomiichuk V, Fleischhammer J, Molliqaj G, Warda J, Alaid A, von Eckardstein K, et al. Robotic versus fluoroscopy-guided pedicle screw insertion for metastatic spinal disease: A matched-cohort comparison. Neurosurgical Focus. 2017;**42**(5):E13

[24] Keric N, Eum DJ, Afghanyar F, Rachwal-Czyzewicz I, Renovanz M, Conrad J, et al. Evaluation of surgical strategy of conventional vs. percutaneous robot-assisted spinal trans-pedicular instrumentation in spondylodiscitis. Journal of Robotic Surgery. 2017;**11**(1):17-25

[25] Keric N, Doenitz C, Haj A, Rachwal-Czyzewicz I, Renovanz M, Wesp DMA, et al. Evaluation of robot-guided minimally invasive implantation of 2067 pedicle screws. Neurosurgical Focus. 2017;**42**(5):E11

[26] Alaid A, von Eckardstein K, Smoll NR, Solomiichuk V, Rohde V, Martinez R, et al. Robot guidance for percutaneous minimally invasive placement of pedicle screws for pyogenic spondylodiscitis is associated with lower rates of wound breakdown compared to conventional fluoroscopy-guided instrumentation. Neurosurgical Review. 2018;**41**(2):489-496

[27] Kim HJ, Jung WI, Chang BS, Lee CK, Kang KT, Yeom JS. A prospective, randomized, controlled trial of robot-assisted vs freehand pedicle screw fixation in spine surgery. International Journal of Medical Robotics and Computer Assisted Surgery. 2017;**13**(e1779)

[28] Roser F, Tatagiba M, Maier G. Spinal robotics: Current applications and future perspectives. Neurosurgery. 2013;**72**(Suppl 1):12-18

[29] Ringel F, Stuer C, Reinke A, Preuss A, Behr M, Auer F, et al. Accuracy of robot-assisted placement of lumbar and sacral pedicle screws: A prospective randomized comparison to conventional freehand screw implantation. Spine. 2012;**37**(8):E496-E501

[30] Hyun SJ, Kim KJ, Jahng TA, Kim HJ. Minimally invasive robotic versus open fluoroscopic-guided

spinal instrumented fusions: A randomized controlled trial. Spine. 2017;**42**(6):353-358

[31] Park SM, Kim HJ, Lee SY, Chang BS, Lee CK, Yeom JS. Radiographic and clinical outcomes of robot-assisted posterior pedicle screw fixation: Two-year results from a randomized controlled trial. Yonsei Medical Journal. 2018;**59**(3):438-444

[32] Lonjon N, Chan-Seng E, Costalat V, Bonnafoux B, Vassal M, Boetto J. Robot-assisted spine surgery: Feasibility study through a prospective case-matched analysis. European Spine Journal. 2016;**25**(3):947-955

[33] Huntsman KT, Ahrendtsen LA, Riggleman JR, Ledonio CG. Robotic-assisted navigated minimally invasive pedicle screw placement in the first 100 cases at a single institution. Journal of Robotic Surgery. 2019

[34] Bederman SS, Hahn P, Colin V, Kiester PD, Bhatia NN. Robotic guidance for S2-alar-iliac screws in spinal deformity correction. Clinical Spine Surgery. 2017;**30**(1):E49-E53

[35] Hu X, Lieberman IH. Robotic-guided sacro-pelvic fixation using S2 alar-iliac screws: Feasibility and accuracy. European Spine Journal. 2017;**26**(3):720-725

[36] Hyun SJ, Kim KJ, Jahng TA. S2 alar iliac screw placement under robotic guidance for adult spinal deformity patients: Technical note. European Spine Journal. 2017;**26**(8):2198-2203

[37] Laratta JL, Shillingford JN, Lombardi JM, Alrabaa RG, Benkli B, Fischer C, et al. Accuracy of S2 alar-iliac screw placement under robotic guidance. Spine Deformity. 2018;**6**(2):130-136

[38] Shillingford JN, Laratta JL, Park PJ, Lombardi JM, Tuchman A, Saifi C, et al. Human versus robot: A propensity-matched analysis of the accuracy of free hand versus robotic guidance for placement of S2 alar-iliac (S2AI) screws. Spine. 2018;**43**(21):E1297-EE304

[39] Vaccaro AR, Zeiller SC, Hulbert RJ, Anderson PA, Harris M, Hedlund R, et al. The thoracolumbar injury severity score: A proposed treatment algorithm. Journal of Spinal Disorders & Techniques. 2005;**18**(3):209-215

[40] Stull JD, Mangan JJ, Vaccaro AR, Schroeder GD. Robotic guidance in minimally invasive spine surgery: A review of recent literature and commentary on a developing technology. Current Reviews in Musculoskeletal Medicine. 2019;**12**(2):245-251

[41] Kim HJ, Lee SH, Chang BS, Lee CK, Lim TO, Hoo LP, et al. Monitoring the quality of robot-assisted pedicle screw fixation in the lumbar spine by using a cumulative summation test. Spine. 2015;**40**(2):87-94

[42] Fan Y, Du J, Zhang J, Liu S, Xue X, Huang Y, et al. Comparison of accuracy of pedicle screw insertion among 4 guided technologies in spine surgery. Medical Science Monitor. 2017;**23**:5960-5968

[43] Marcus HJ, Cundy TP, Nandi D, Yang GZ, Darzi A. Robot-assisted and fluoroscopy-guided pedicle screw placement: A systematic review. European Spine Journal. 2014;**23**(2):291-297

[44] Knez D, Likar B, Pernus F, Vrtovec T. Computer-assisted screw size and insertion trajectory planning for pedicle screw placement surgery. IEEE Transactions on Medical Imaging. 2016;**35**(6):1420-1430

[45] Knez D, Nahle IS, Vrtovec T, Parent S, Kadoury S, editors. Computer-assisted pedicle screw placement

planning: Towards clinical practice. In: 2018 IEEE 15th International Symposium on Biomedical Imaging (ISBI 2018); 4-7 April 2018

[46] Vijayan R, De Silva T, Han R, Zhang X, Uneri A, Doerr S, et al. Automatic pedicle screw planning using atlas-based registration of anatomy and reference trajectories. Physics in Medicine and Biology. 2019

Chapter 2

Innovations in the Surgery of Cerebral Aneurysms: Enhanced Visualization, Perfusion, and Function Monitoring

Oriela Rustemi, Alessandro Della Puppa and Alba Scerrati

Abstract

Surgery of cerebral aneurysms has evolved over the years. Advances regard enhanced intraoperative visualization and monitoring of both function and perfusion. Technological assistance used in oncological or skull base surgery, such as intraoperative neurophysiological monitoring (IONM) or endoscopy, now adopt to vascular surgery. Intraoperative indocyanine green video angiography (ICG-VA) and techniques for its interpretation (squeezing maneuver; entrapment sign), endoscopes, and exoscopes increase visualization. Flow evaluation by microflow probe permits perfusion monitoring; IONM allows functional monitoring. Bypasses replace flow in complex aneurysm cases. Pre-, intra-, and postoperative imaging and flow measurement techniques help in donor selection and follow-up. Despite some progression in the aneurysm clips, the principle has not changed. Innovation and even change of principle in aneurysm exclusion might be desirable. Basic research in aneurysm wall and flow dynamics might in the future change the paradigms of cerebral aneurysm treatment.

Keywords: aneurysm surgery, cerebral aneurysm, bypass, clipping, vascular surgery, indocyanine green video angiography, flow measurement, neurophysiological monitoring, perivascular flow probe, endoscope

1. Introduction

The advent of endovascular treatment determined the crisis of cerebral aneurysm surgery. Endovascular therapy is less invasive and its progression is rapid. Industries' interests and investments potentiate the technological endovascular advancements. Surgical treatment by clipping of intracranial aneurysms is durable and stable in time. There are advances in making surgical treatment safer and offering treatment to the more complicated cases, not amenable to endovascular therapy. Advances and investments in the surgery of cerebral aneurysms are less deafening in the last decade. However, some silent innovative advances are made over the years. Here we present innovations in cerebral aneurysm surgery.

2. Enhanced intraoperative visualization: intraoperative indocyanine green video angiography (ICG-VA) principle and implantation in vascular neurosurgery

Indocyanine green (ICG) is a near-infrared (NIR) fluorescent dye initially approved by the Food and Drug Administration (FDA) in 1956 for the evaluation of the cardiocirculatory and liver function. FDA extended the approval for ophthalmic angiography in 1975. Nowadays, ICG fluorescence is routinely used in ophthalmology for the visualization of the retinal microcirculation. A specific optical setup for near-infrared (NIR) light is necessary for the visualization of the ICG fluorescence. The development of an ICG angiography new system allowed further implementation for the intraoperative visualization of the tissue perfusion in general surgery.

Raabe et al. gave a substantial contribution by implementing ICG angiography use in vascular neurosurgery [1].

The absorption peak of ICG is 805 nm, while the emission peak is 835 nm. Within these two peaks, the endogenous tissue chromophore absorption is low.

NIR light penetrates the tissue from several millimeters to a few centimeters. ICG is injected intravenously, and it bounds in 1–2 s predominantly to globulins (α1-lipoproteins). In the absence of vascular permeability damage, ICG bound to globulins remains intravascular. ICG has a plasma half-life of 3–4 min. It is only excreted by the liver with no metabolization.

Raabe et al. used a laser-fluorescence imaging device (IC-View; Pulsion Medical Systems AG, Munich, Germany), consisting of a NIR laser light source (0.16 W, $\lambda = 780$ nm) and a NIR-sensitive digital camcorder.

ICG was injected intravenously in a bolus (standard dose of 25 mg dissolved in 5 ml of water). ICG fluorescence was induced by the NIR light emitted by the laser light source. The digital video camera with optical filtering recorded only the ICG-induced fluorescence signal.

The near-infrared filter was commercially available for surgical microscopes routinely used in neurosurgery, and ICG-VA could be applied in vascular neurosurgery.

For example, intraoperative ICG-VA could be performed using a surgical microscope (OPMI® PenteroTM, The Carl Zeiss Co., Oberkochen, Germany) equipped with a microscope-integrated near-infrared ICG-VA (Carl Zeiss, Infrared 800TM, Meditec, Germany). ICG is injected intravenously in a bolus of 25 mg dissolved in 5 ml of water, and the operating field is illuminated with near-infrared light. Real-time angiographic images are visualized on a video screen and recorded. The images can be replayed. Only the illuminated field is recorded. ICG can be injected multiple times during surgery; thus ICG-VA is repeatable.

3. ICG-VA for accessing aneurysm occlusion after clipping

After Raabe's first report [1], ICG-VA gradually became routinely used in aneurysm surgery. It is used after aneurysm clipping to access whether the aneurysm occlusion is complete. Catheter angiography is the gold standard for cerebral aneurysm diagnosis [2] and for confirming aneurysm occlusion. However, intraoperative catheter angiography requires a programmed setup; is invasive, expensive, and time-consuming, and requires a well-trained staff. It is reserved to particular complicated cases, and it is not intraoperatively routinely used in the surgery of intracranial aneurysms. Furthermore, the time required for an intraoperative angiogram may be sufficient for the establishment of irreversible ischemia. Postoperative residual aneurysms after clipping are reported in a variable range from 4 to 19%

of cases [3–10]. ICG-VA is fast, easily used, and not invasive. It allows immediate assessment of the aneurysm occlusion after clipping, and permits whether necessary clip repositioning or further clip positioning. Although, ICG-VA is inferior to catheter angiography in assessing aneurysm complete occlusion, it is intraoperatively easily used in the cases where intraoperative catheter angiography would not be used routinely. It does not substitute postoperative neuroradiological control of aneurysm complete occlusion but allows to have higher postoperative occlusion rates. Postoperative catheter angiography remains the gold standard for assessment of aneurysm occlusion. Generally, intraoperative ICG-VA is used to access clipping after apparent complete occlusion under the microscope light. Della Puppa et al. showed that despite apparent complete occlusion under microscope visualization, ICG-VA revealed unexpected residual aneurysms in 9% [11]. Roessler et al. in a study of 295 aneurysms clipped with the use of ICG-VA showed an intraoperative clip modification rate of 15% based on ICG-VA data [12]. Thus, ICG-VA is a complementary tool that increases aneurysm occlusion rate, but it does not substitute postoperative digital subtraction angiography (DSA) for the detection of aneurysm remnants [13]. Intraoperative aneurysm puncture, or opening whenever possible, remains the most reliable intraoperative measure to assess complete occlusion.

4. Tools to improve ICG-VA interpretation

Different factors can determine false-negative or false-positive ICG-VA findings. Arteriosclerosis and wall thickening at the clipping site influence false-negative ICG-VA findings [14]. Repeated ICG can determine false-positive results. Also, a small remnant detected in ICG can undergo spontaneous thrombosis and thus may not present a real residual.

4.1 Squeezing maneuver

ICG-VA despite improvement of aneurysm occlusions rate can also show deceptive false-negative results. Della Puppa et al. described a surgical simple maneuver to detect false-negative ICG-VA results after clipping of a cerebral aneurysm [15]. The squeezing maneuver consists of a gentle pinch with bipolar/Cushing bayonet forceps of the dome of a clipped aneurysm when ICG-VA documents its apparent exclusion.

The maneuver is performed during the same ICG injection to confirm the aneurysm exclusion. It is considered positive when, after an initial ICG-VA shows the aneurysm exclusion, a gentle pinch of the slack aneurysm dome with a bipolar or Cushing bayonet forceps under ICG-VA visualization causes the prompt dyeing of the sac, suggesting that the aneurysm is still filling up. The maneuver is considered negative when, after pinching of the clipped dome, the sac does not fill up. The puncture and opening of the sac can confirm whether a flow is still filling the aneurysm. The squeezing maneuver can depict ICG-VA false-negative results.

This permits to readjust the clip or position a second clip to completely exclude the aneurysm during the same procedure. Calcification/atheroma of the wall/neck was predictive of a positive maneuver (P = 0.001). This is consistent with Gekka et al. findings several years later, which report false-negative ICG-VA results in atherosclerosis and wall thickening at the clipping site [14].

4.2 ICG entrapment sign

ICG-VA can also show false-positive results, if misinterpreted. When ICG is injected before the final aneurysm clipping, the dye might be entrapped within the sac by the clip's blades, which would obstacle the dye washout. ICG-VA would show the dye entrapped in the sac. An erroneous interpretation of the data would be to consider the aneurysm unsecured. Della Puppa et al. introduced the ICG entrapment sign as the detection under infrared light of ICG remnants sequestered in the dome [16]. ICG entrapment sign detects dye stasis, and not active filling. It is considered a sign of aneurysm occlusion in the setting of ICG injection prior to final clipping. This may happen if ICG is injected prior to clipping for visualization of perforating arteries near to the sac or detection of atheromas of the neck/dome. This happens more commonly after clip repositioning based on ICG indication.

The squeezing maneuver can detect a false-negative ICG-VA (an unsecured aneurysm despite apparent occlusion after ICG), whereas the ICG entrapment sign can detect a false-positive ICV-VA result (a secured aneurysm under infrared light, despite ICG-VA showing dye).

5. Other ICG-VA uses

5.1 Transdural application

ICG-VA can be used before dural opening in vascular arteriovenous malformations or fistulas to optimize the exposure of the malformation, perform a safe dural opening, and identify dural vascular connections of the lesion [17]. The cases where transdural ICG can help in aneurysm surgery are very rare. These are the cases of distal cortical, generally distal middle cerebral artery (M4) aneurysms. In a case of M4 ruptured aneurysm, ICG-VA allowed transdural aneurysm visualization [18]. This is particularly helpful in an emergency setting, when neuronavigation is not available, to localize the aneurysm and avoid damage while opening the dura.

5.2 Transoptic aneurysm visualization

Other exceptional ICG-VA applications reported are the transoptic aneurysm visualization and occlusion confirmation in a case of an optic splitting aneurysm [19]. An ophthalmic artery aneurysm medially and superiorly projecting, suspicious for an under optic growth, underwent surgery. Initially the aneurysm was not visible. ICG-VA permitted the transoptic aneurysm visualization and after clipping final occlusion.

ICG-VA application was extended in other pathologies [20–26].

5.3 Flow measurement by microflow probe: principle and implementation in neurosurgery

Vascular micro-Dopplers are used in cerebral aneurysm surgery to indicate the flow velocity. They are easy to use and give the surgeon an acoustic signal feedback. The flow velocity is used as a surrogate of the flow quantity. Flow velocity is not the most reliable indicator for flow. Flow quantity is the most reliable flow measure.

Till the 1990s, the intraoperative ultrasonic blood flow probes have been used to quantitatively measure flow only in cardiac, vascular, and transplant surgery. Charbel et al. in the University of Illinois at Chicago first reported in 1997 the implantation of the ultrasonic perivascular micro blood flow probes in the clipping of cerebral aneurysms [27–31].

The first transit time flowmeters were described in 1962 and 1964 [32, 33]. Limitations in estimating vessel diameter, vessel misalignment, and an unstable zero calibration prevented medical applications [34]. In 1978 Drost et al. presented the theoretical basis for a flowmeter based on the transit time technique [35, 36]. The transit time flowmeter was introduced in 1983 [36].

The transit time blood volume flowmeter gives a direct measurement of volume flow through the acoustic window of its implanted sensor, independent of flow profile. In contrast, earlier Doppler and transit time ultrasonic flowmeters sense blood velocity, which makes volume flow measurements critically dependent on vessel diameter [35, 36].

The transonic perivascular flow-measuring device includes an electronic flow detection unit with enhanced frequency resolution and volume flow-sensing perivascular probes (Transonic Medical Flowmeter; Transonic Systems, Inc., Ithaca, NY, USA). The perivascular flow probes are manufactured in 1.5, 2, and 3 mm diameter and can be used to measure the average flow volume (mL/min) instantaneously in cerebral vessels.

The flowmeter uses ultrasonic transit time principle to sense liquid volume flow in vessels independent of flow velocity, hematocrit, and turbulence.

The electronic flow-detecting unit is a line-powered flowmeter that automatically identifies the scaling factor and individual calibration factor of the flow probe connected to it. The flow sensors are connected to the flow-detecting unit via a flexible cable.

The ultrasonic transducers transmit ultrasound which helps to sense the volume of blood flowing through the blood vessel in which the sensor is applied.

The flow probe consists of a probe body which houses two ultrasonic transducers and a fixed acoustic reflector. The transducer is positioned around the blood vessel, and then the flow in that vessel is displayed in the digital form. The flowmeter derives an accurate measure of the "transit time," which is the time the wave of ultrasound has taken to travel from one transducer to the other [28].

Practically, a portion of the vessel of interest is dissected from the arachnoid, and the probe is hooked around the vessel under saline irrigation.

The flow appears as a digital display on the detection unit and is registered as positive or negative dependent on the direction of flow in relation to the orientation of the probe. The flow is detected as the volume (mL/min), and the flow volume over time of recording diagram can be printed.

5.4 Flow measurement by microflow probe: application in aneurysm surgery

Quantitative blood flow measurement became essential in blood flow preservation to avoid postoperative ischemic complication in cerebral aneurysm surgery. Amin-Hanjani et al. proposed a baseline evaluation of blood flow in the vessels at risk of flow compromise after clipping (generally the efferent arteries, distal to the aneurysm) and a second flow evaluation of the same vessels after clipping [31]. A reduction of the flow greater than 25% of baseline was considered at risk for ischemic complications, and the clip was repositioned. The data was reproduced by other studies [11, 37, 38]. Flow measurement by microflow probe was also used in other cerebrovascular diseases [39–42].

6. Intraoperative neurophysiological monitoring IONM

IONM routinely used in oncological surgery, over the years, has become essential also in vascular surgery to avoid ischemic complications. Monitoring includes bilateral upper and lower limb motor evoked potentials (MEPs) and somatosensory evoked potentials (SSEPs). Generally, in aneurysm surgery, MEPs are monitored by transcranial electric stimulation, rather than by direct cortical mapping, because the motor area is not routinely exposed during standard pterional approaches for anterior circulation aneurysms, and it is never exposed with mini invasive approaches. Direct electrical cortical stimulation might also increase the risk of epileptic seizures. For MEP monitoring transcranial electric stimulation is made by electrodes positioned at C1 and C2 according to the 10–20 International System (IS). These electrodes continuously stimulate the motor area during surgery by train stimuli (the pulse trains used are different according to the users; there are reported 4–8 pulse trains) [37, 43]. MEPs are recorded by subcutaneous needle electrodes from the abductor pollicis brevis and abductor hallucis muscles. The baseline MEPs are recorded at the beginning of the surgery, and it is found a compromise with the surgeon between continuous MEP recording and the movements caused by the stimuli tolerated by the surgeon for the dissection and clipping procedure. To avoid false-negative results on MEPs, the stimulus applied for MEP acquisition should be minimal not to activate the distal motor pathways [44]. To avoid false-positive results, brain shift due to the cerebrospinal loss after cisternal opening should be considered.

The reduction of 50% in MEP amplitude or MEP disappearance is considered as an alarm criterion. The surgeon changes the strategy to tempt to recover the MEPs. Temporary clipping is interrupted, or the definitive clip is released. The arterial blood pressure may be increased; local irrigation with saline and papaverine may be tempted. The surgical procedure is temporarily stopped, whenever it is possible (the aneurysm is not intraoperatively ruptured, or it is not opened by the surgeon) to permit the MEPs to recover. The MEP deterioration can be reversible, when the MEPs return to more than 50% of baseline amplitude.

Another methodology of MEP monitoring is by direct cortical stimulation.

Upper limb SSEPs are recorded from C3 and C4 by electrically stimulating the contralateral median nerve at the wrist. Lower limbs are recorded by electric stimulation of the contralateral tibial nerve at the medial malleolus. Recordings from Cz′ and Fz are made according to the 10–20 International System [37].

A total intravenous anesthesia (TIVA) is used. Neuromuscular blockers are not used during surgery, unless extremely necessary. Muscle relaxants are used only for endotracheal intubation.

An early experimental study by Branston et al. in 1974 showed that there is a failure of neuronal function in the cortex when the local blood flow falls below about 16 ml/100 g/min. This failure becomes manifest as a progressive reduction in the amplitude of the surface recorded SSEP, and this results in the abolition of the SSEPs if the flow is below about 12 ml/l00 g/min. There is a close relationship between reduced cerebral blood flow (CBF: 12–16 ml/100 g/min) and a reduction in SSEP amplitude or SSEP abolition [45].

MEP monitoring has higher diagnostic accuracy than SSEPs in predicting the occurrence of a postoperative neurological deficit [46].

Li et al. analyzed 92 patients operated for cerebral aneurysms that showed intraoperative MEP deterioration. They found that a MEP deterioration duration greater than or equal to 13 min in intracranial aneurysm surgery was significantly associated with postoperative motor deficits [43].

7. Awake surgery in the surgery of intracranial aneurysms

The principles of neuro-oncological monitoring are being gradually transferred to cerebral aneurysm surgery. In neuro-oncological surgery, the best way to monitor the neurological and neurophysiological function is by awake surgery. Awake surgery of cerebral aneurysms is controversial for the potential consequences of intraoperative aneurysm rupture. Intraoperative aneurysm rupture does not impact the clinical outcome. This would not be true if the clipping was performed in awake surgery. However, in selected case of clipping of the aneurysms of the dominant hemisphere, the monitoring of the language function and thus awake surgery would be useful. Abdulrauf et al. reported awake surgery in 30 unruptured cerebral aneurysms [47]. In three patients the strategy affected the outcome, since the removal of the temporary clipping determined the reversal of the clinical neurological and neurophysiological changes. One patient developed a neurological damage depending on the clipping, but that could not be reversed by the clip repositioning. Three patients developed hemiparesis without changes in MEPs; thus they were false negatives. The important was the visual testing after final clipping in four patients with internal carotid artery ophthalmic segment aneurysms, and one of these patients required repositioning of the clip. Three patients underwent an intraoperative vessel occlusion test, since the vessel occlusion was part of the permanent treatment of the aneurysm.

8. Blind spot avoidance and mini invasive approaches

8.1 Endoscopic-assisted clipping

The endoscope is mainly used as assistance during microsurgical clipping of intracranial aneurysms. The endoscopic-assisted microsurgery has been promoted by the father of the keyhole approaches Perneczky and by Fries [48]. The endoscope can be used for inspection before clipping; also clipping under endoscopic view and post clipping evaluation to observe the perforator integrity can be performed [49]. The endoscope allows the visualization of the blind spots to the microscope, allows thus the vision around corners, and enhances the visualization. It can potentially ameliorate the quality of treatment. The microscope enables vision in a straight line, while the endoscope enables the visualization of angles. The endoscope can be complementary to the microscope. However, the surgeon must be familiar with the endoscope use, not to cause iatrogenic damage [50].

8.2 Endoscopic ICG-VA

Endoscopic ICG-VA is an important development that combines the benefits of the vision behind the corners of endoscopy and the vessel visualization of ICG-VA [51]. The combination of both is particularly important for the visualization of the perforating arteries hidden in blind spots.

8.3 Pure endoscopic transcranial or endonasal

Purely endoscopic approach to cerebral aneurysms is a potential method in its very beginning. There are case reports of endonasal clipping of aneurysms and of endoscopic transcranial pure approaches.

Radovanovic reports a cadaveric study of a purely endoscopic transpterional port craniotomy to access lesions involving the cavernous sinus and the anterolateral skull base [52]. In the illustration videos, the author includes clipping of a middle cerebral artery aneurysm through this approach. There are also strictly selected case reports or small series of endoscopic endonasal clipping of anterior circulation aneurysms [53]. Other case reports regard the pure endoscopic endonasal transclival approach for clipping of posterior circulation aneurysms [54]. These minimally invasive approaches constitute very limited experiences, and they need very deep expertise; otherwise they become dangerous. Safety must never be sacrificed for achieving minimal invasiveness.

8.4 Exoscope

Exoscopes are projected to combine the benefits of neurosurgical microscopes and endoscopes. With the exoscope, the surgeon looks at the monitor while operating, and the entire surgical team has the same view as the primary surgeon. The 3D 4K-HD exoscopes have favorable ergonomics to visualize angles maintaining the surgeon's comfort, maneuverability, and immersive visual experience. The assistant positioning relative to the surgeon can be problematic during surgery. ORBEYE (Olympus, Tokyo, Japan) exoscope has been used in aneurysm surgery with reported excellent visualization of the arterial tree [55], but with a subjective disadvantage in the visualization of bleeding tissue particularly in the muscle or white matter [56]. This new technology is proposed with advantages and limits, and time will tell its exact role in the future.

9. Perforating artery evaluation

The perforating arteries are small twigs of the main cerebral arteries that irrorate the paramedian region of the brainstem, the diencephalon, the basal ganglia, and the internal capsule [57]. Commonly, the perforators are small vessels of less than 1 mm in diameter, except for some lenticulostriate arteries (LSAs) and Heubner arteries larger than 1 mm. They may be multiple and sometimes anastomose. Although the same territory can be supplied by multiple perforators, the consequence of the occlusion of a perforator is unpredictable and more often than not results in a neurological deficit. Perforator infarction was shown as an independent risk factor of poor functional outcome in a series of anterior communicating aneurysms [58]. In the surgery of cerebral aneurysms, it is essential to preserve the perforating arteries. While the flow preservation of a larger artery is easier and eventually the flow can be replaced by revascularization, the perforator damage is more feared and less predictable. The monitoring of the perforators is fundamental. ICG-VA has the advantage of being able to visualize the perforating arteries. As a speculation, it is assumed that flowmetry and SSEPs account for the cortical gray matter function while the MEPs for the subcortical white matter function. Thus, MEPs can be used to evaluate the perforating artery function, and ICG-VA allows their visualization along with endoscopes, exoscopes, and endoscopic ICG-VA that permit the vision behind blind points.

10. Complementary tools

None of the tools described is superior to the others, and their role in improving clinical results in aneurysm surgery is complementary. Della Puppa et al. have described the complementary role of enhanced visualization with ICG-VA and maneuvers and signs to better interpret the data, along with monitoring of function (IONM) and perfusion (flowmetry) [37].

11. Quantitative magnetic resonance angiography and donor selection in bypass surgery for flow replacement

Quantitative magnetic resonance angiography (QMRA) is an MRA that permits blood flow quantification of the major cerebral vessels [59, 60]. QMRA is implemented with a commercially available software called Noninvasive Optimal Vessel Analysis (NOVA) (VasSol, Inc., Chicago, Illinois). MRA creates the cerebral vascular tree. A double-oblique scan is performed using a gated two-dimensional phase-contrast MRA imaged perpendicular to the vessel of interest axis. The software generates a flow report with the mean volumetric flow rate (mL/min) of the vessels of interest. QMRA data have been validated in vivo and have shown proportional differences, around 10% to direct transit time flow measurements [60]. QMRA is reported to be used preoperatively to evaluate the flow of the major vessels in patients with cerebral aneurysm that would require a bypass, when vessel sacrifice is needed to treat the aneurysm [42]. Intraoperatively a flow-based algorithm can be used to determine the flow needed to replace the flow sacrificed. Transit time flow measurements are used for intraoperative measurements. These measurements indicate which is the more appropriate donor graft to be used for the anastomosis. This methodology has shown that superficial temporal artery is often sufficient to replace flow, which renders the surgery easier than using vein or radial artery grafts. QMRA is used in follow-up to detect the bypass flow. The hemisphere flows are calculated and are maintained over time. Details of the algorithm used for calculation of the flow needed to be replaced and the donor flow potential can be found in the paper by Rustemi et al. [42].

12. Intracranial-intracranial bypass

Lawton has rendered popular the intracranial-intracranial (IC-IC) bypass for flow replacement in complex aneurysms [61]. This type of bypass, although more elegant, has several pitfalls and requires very experienced surgeons. IC-IC bypass puts at dangers both the donor and receiving territories. The anastomosis is deep and more difficult to be performed. However, in selected cases and experienced hands, it represents an advancement.

13. Sutureless excimer laser-assisted nonocclusive anastomosis (SELANA)

The ELANA has been developed for intracranial bypass without the need for temporary recipient occlusion. A sutureless variant of the ELANA—the SELANA slide—showed a preclinical success and clinical application started. Unfortunately, it was not shown suitable for clinical applications [62].

14. Future prospective

Many technological innovations now assist the surgeon in the treatment of cerebral aneurysms. Also, different clips are used over the years. However, the clip principle has not changed. A change in occlusion strategy, based on principles other than clipping, might be desirable for the future. There is space for new ideas and new principles. The basic research studies for cerebral aneurysms are focused on wall analysis and flow stimulations. If advances will become more solid, in the future, cerebral aneurysms will not need neurosurgeons or neuroendovascular radiologists.

15. Conclusions

Surgery of cerebral aneurysms has advanced over the years. Innovations are rapid in this technological era. Many innovations are now routinely used in the clinical practice; others will be soon implemented. The technological innovations currently used in the surgery of cerebral aneurysms are summarized in this chapter. The comprehension of the biology and pathology might in the future render the aneurysm a medical disease.

Conflict of interest

Nothing to declare.

Acronyms and abbreviations

IONM	intraoperative neurophysiological monitoring
ICG-VA	indocyanine green video angiography
ICG	indocyanine green
NIR	near-infrared
FDA	Food and Drug Administration
M4	distal middle cerebral artery
MEPs	motor evoked potentials
SSEPs	somatosensory evoked potentials
IS	International System
TIVA	total intravenous anesthesia
CBF	cerebral blood flow
LSAs	lenticulostriate arteries
QMRA	quantitative magnetic resonance angiography
NOVA	Noninvasive Optimal Vessel Analysis
IC-IC	intracranial-intracranial
ELANA	excimer laser-assisted nonocclusive anastomosis
SELANA	sutureless ELANA

Author details

Oriela Rustemi[1*], Alessandro Della Puppa[2,3] and Alba Scerrati[4]

1 Department of Neurosurgery, San Bortolo Hospital, Vicenza, Italy

2 Department of Neurosurgery, University of Florence, Florence, Italy

3 Department of Neurosurgery, Neuroscience, Psychology, Pharmacology, and Child Health, University of Florence, Careggi, Florence, Italy

4 Department of Neurosurgery, S. Anna University Hospital, Ferrara, Italy

*Address all correspondence to: orielarustemi@libero.it

References

[1] Raabe A, Beck J, Gerlach R, Zimmermann M, Seifert V. Near-infrared indocyanine green video angiography: A new method for intraoperative assessment of vascular flow. Neurosurgery. 2003;**52**:132-139; discussion 139

[2] Rustemi O, Alaraj A, Shakur SF, Orning JL, Du X, Aletich VA, et al. Detection of unruptured intracranial aneurysms on noninvasive imaging. Is there still a role for digital subtraction angiography? Surgical Neurology International. 2015;**6**:175. DOI: 10.4103/2152-7806.170029

[3] Alexander TD, Macdonald RL, Weir B, Kowalczuk A. Intraoperative angiography in cerebral aneurysm surgery: A prospective study of 100 craniotomies. Neurosurgery. 1996;**39**:10-18

[4] Drake C, Allcock J. Postoperative angiography and the slipped clip. Journal of Neurosurgery. 1973;**39**:683-689

[5] Feuerberg I, Lindquist C, Lindqvist M, Steiner L. Natural history of postoperative aneurysm rests. Journal of Neurosurgery. 1987;**66**:30-34

[6] Macdonald RL, Wallace MC, Kestle JR. Role of angiography following aneurysm surgery. Journal of Neurosurgery. 1993;**79**:826-832

[7] Proust F, Hannequin D, Langlois O, Freger P, Creissard P. Causes of morbidity and mortality after ruptured aneurysm surgery in a series of 230 patients. The importance of control angiography. Stroke. 1995;**26**:1553-1557

[8] Rauzzino MJ, Quinn CM, Fisher WS. Angiography after aneurysm surgery: Indications for selective angiography. Surgical Neurology. 1998;**49**:32-40

[9] Samson D, Hodosh R, Reid W, Beyer CW, Clark WK. Risk of intracranial aneurysm surgery in the good grade patient: Early versus late operation. Neurosurgery. 1979;**5**:422-426

[10] Suzuki J, Kwak R, Katakura R. Review of incompletely occluded surgically treated cerebral aneurysms. Surgical Neurology. 1980;**13**:306-310

[11] Della Puppa A, Volpin F, Gioffre G, Rustemi O, Troncon I, Scienza R. Microsurgical clipping of intracranial aneurysms assisted by green indocyanine videoangiography (ICG-VA) and ultrasonic perivascular microflow probe measurement. Clinical Neurology and Neurosurgery. 2014;**116**:35-40. DOI: 10.1016/j.clineuro.2013.11.004

[12] Roessler K, Krawagna M, Dörfler A, Buchfelder M, Ganslandt O. Essentials in intraoperative indocyanine green videoangiography assessment for intracranial aneurysm surgery: Conclusions from 295 consecutively clipped aneurysms and review of the literature. Neurosurgical Focus. 2014;**36**:E7. DOI: 10.3171/2013.11.FOCUS13475

[13] Riva M, Amin-Hanjani S, Giussani C, De Witte O, Bruneau M. Indocyanine green videoangiography in aneurysm surgery: Systematic review and meta-analysis. Neurosurgery. 2018;**83**:166-180. DOI: 10.1093/neuros/nyx387

[14] Gekka M, Nakayama N, Uchino H, Houkin K. Factors influencing cerebral aneurysm obliteration and reliability of indocyanine green video-angiography. Acta Neurochirurgica. 2018;**160**:269-276. DOI: 10.1007/s00701-017-3379-6

[15] Della Puppa A, Rustemi O, Rossetto M, Gioffrè G, Munari M, Charbel FT, et al. The “squeezing

maneuver" in microsurgical clipping of intracranial aneurysms assisted by indocyanine green videoangiography. Neurosurgery. 2014;**10**:208-212; discussion 212-203. DOI: 10.1227/NEU.0000000000000334

[16] Della Puppa A, Rustemi O, Scienza R. The "ICG Entrapment Sign" in cerebral aneurysm surgery assisted by indocyanine green videoangiography. World Neurosurgery. 2017;**97**:287-291. DOI: 10.1016/j.wneu.2016.10.011

[17] Della Puppa A, Rustemi O, Gioffrè G, Causin F, Scienza R. Transdural indocyanine green video-angiography of vascular malformations. Acta Neurochirurgica. 2014;**156**:1761-1767. DOI: 10.1007/s00701-014-2164-z

[18] Rustemi O, Scienza R, Della Puppa A. Indocyanine green videoangiography application in distal (M4) middle cerebral artery aneurysm surgery. Journal of Neurosurgical Sciences. 2017;**61**:351-354. DOI: 10.23736/S0390-5616.16.03271-9

[19] Rustemi O, Cester G, Causin F, Scienza R, Della Puppa A. Indocyanine green videoangiography transoptic visualization and clipping confirmation of an optic splitting ophthalmic artery aneurysm. World Neurosurgery. 2016;**90**:705.e5-705.e8. DOI: 10.1016/j.wneu.2016.03.010

[20] Della Puppa A, d'Avella E, Volpin F, Rustemi O, Gioffre' G, Scienza R. Indocyanine green videoangiography (ICG-VA) in parasagittal meningiomas surgery. Considerations on veins management and brain function preservation. Acta Neurochirurgica. 2013;**155**:1475-1476. DOI: 10.1007/s00701-013-1784-z

[21] Della Puppa A, Rustemi O, Gioffrè G. Is the intra-operative application of indocyanine green effective in retro-orbital surgery? Acta Neurochirurgica. 2014;**156**:1419-1420. DOI: 10.1007/s00701-014-2001-4

[22] Della Puppa A, Rustemi O, Gioffrè G, Rolma G, Grandis M, Munari M, et al. Application of indocyanine green video angiography in parasagittal meningioma surgery. Neurosurgical Focus. 2014;**36**:E13. DOI: 10.3171/2013.12.FOCUS13385

[23] Rustemi O, Scienza R, Della Puppa A. ICG-VA application in subtemporal transtentorial treatment of a Cognard V dural arteriovenous fistula. Neurosurg Focus. 2016;**40**(Video Suppl 1):V7. DOI: 10.3171/2016.1.FocusVid.15423

[24] Rustemi O, Scienza R, Della Puppa A. Intra-operative devascularization of petroclival meningiomas by ICG-VA-guided Bernasconi & Cassinari artery identification. Acta Neurochirurgica. 2016;**158**:427-428. DOI: 10.1007/s00701-016-2704-9

[25] Rustemi O, Scienza R, Della Puppa A. Utility of indocyanine green videoangiography in subcortical arteriovenous malformation resection. Neurosurgical Focus. 2017;**43**(Video Suppl 1):V10. DOI: 10.3171/2017.7.FocusVid.1774

[26] Scerrati A, Della Pepa GM, Conforti G, Sabatino G, Puca A, Albanese A, et al. Indocyanine green video-angiography in neurosurgery: A glance beyond vascular applications. Clinical Neurology and Neurosurgery. 2014;**124**:106-113. DOI: 10.1016/j.clineuro.2014.06.032

[27] Hoffman WE, Charbel FT, Ausman JI. Cerebral blood flow and metabolic response to etomidate and ischemia. Neurological Research. 1997;**19**:41-44

[28] Charbel FT, Hoffman WE, Misra M, Hannigan K, Ausman JI. Role of a perivascular ultrasonic micro-flow

probe in aneurysm surgery. Neurologia Medico-Chirurgica (Tokyo). 1998;**38**(Suppl):35-38

[29] Charbel FT, Hoffman WE, Misra M, Ostergren L. Ultrasonic perivascular flow probe: Technique and application in neurosurgery. Neurological Research. 1998;**20**:439-442

[30] Charbel FT, Gonzales-Portillo G, Hoffman WE, Ostergren LA, Misra M. Quantitative assessment of vessel flow integrity for aneurysm surgery. Technical note. Journal of Neurosurgery. 1999;**91**:1050-1054

[31] Amin-Hanjani S, Meglio G, Gatto R, Bauer A, Charbel FT. The utility of intraoperative blood flow measurement during aneurysm surgery using an ultrasonic perivascular flow probe. Neurosurgery. 2006;**58**:ONS-305-ONS-312; discussion ONS-312

[32] Franklin DL, Ellis RS, Rushmer RF. Ultrasonic transit time flowmeter. IRE Trans Biomed Eng. 1962:44-49

[33] Plass KG. A new ultrasonic flowmeter for intravascular application. IEEE Transactions on Biomedical Engineering. 1964;**BME-11**:154-156

[34] Lundell A, Bergqvist D, Mattsson E, Nilsson B. Volume blood flow measurements with a transit time flowmeter: An in vivo and in vitro variability and validation study. Clinical Physiology. 1993;**13**:547-557

[35] Drost CJ. Vessel diameter-independent volume flow measurements using ultrasound. Proceedings of San Diego Biomedical Symposium. 1978;**17**:299

[36] Barnes RJ, Comline RS, Dobson A, Drost CJ. An implantable transit-time ultrasonic blood flow-meter. The Journal of Physiology. 1983;**34**:2

[37] Della Puppa A, Rossetto M, Volpin F, Rustemi O, Grego A, Gerardi A, et al. Microsurgical clipping of intracranial aneurysms assisted by neurophysiological monitoring, microvascular flow probe, and ICG-VA: Outcomes and intraoperative data on a multimodal strategy. World Neurosurgery. 2018;**113**:e336-e344. DOI: 10.1016/j.wneu.2018.02.029

[38] Pasqualin A, Meneghelli P, Musumeci A, Della Puppa A, Pavesi G, Pinna G, et al. Intraoperative measurement of arterial blood flow in aneurysm surgery. Acta Neurochirurgica. Supplement. 2018;**129**:43-52. DOI: 10.1007/978-3-319-73739-3_7

[39] Della Puppa A, Scienza R, Rustemi O, Gioffré G. Can the efficacy of indocyanine green videoangiography in cerebral arterio-venous malformations surgery be further improved? Neurosurgery. 2014;**75**:E732-E734. DOI: 10.1227/NEU.0000000000000531

[40] Della Puppa A, Rustemi O, Scienza R. Intraoperative flow measurement by microflow probe during surgery for brain arteriovenous malformations. Neurosurgery. 2015;**11**:268-273. DOI: 10.1227/NEU.0000000000000741

[41] Della Puppa A, Rustemi O, Scienza R. Intraoperative flow measurement by microflow probe during spinal dural arteriovenous fistula surgery. World Neurosurgery. 2016;**89**:413-419. DOI: 10.1016/j.wneu.2016.02.043

[42] Rustemi O, Amin-Hanjani S, Shakur SF, Du X, Charbel FT. Donor selection in flow replacement bypass surgery for cerebral aneurysms: Quantitative analysis of long-term native donor flow sufficiency. Neurosurgery. 2016;**78**:332-341; discussion 341-342. DOI: 10.1227/NEU.0000000000001074

[43] Li Z, Fan X, Wang M, Tao X, Qi L, Ling M, et al. Prediction of postoperative motor deficits using motor evoked potential deterioration duration in intracranial aneurysm surgery. Clinical Neurophysiology. 2019;**130**:707-713. DOI: 10.1016/j.clinph.2019.02.010

[44] Guo L, Gelb AW. The use of motor evoked potential monitoring during cerebral aneurysm surgery to predict pure motor deficits due to subcortical ischemia. Clinical Neurophysiology. 2011;**122**:648-655

[45] Branston NM, Symon L, Crockard HA, Pasztor E. Relationship between the cortical evoked potential and local cortical blood flow following acute middle cerebral artery occlusion in the baboon. Experimental Neurology. 1974;**45**:195-208. DOI: 10.1016/0014-4886(74)90112-5

[46] Thomas B, Guo D. The diagnostic accuracy of evoked potential monitoring techniques during intracranial aneurysm surgery for predicting postoperative ischemic damage: A systematic review and meta-analysis. World Neurosurgery. 2017;**103**:829-840.e3. DOI: 10.1016/j.wneu.2017.04.071

[47] Abdulrauf SI, Vuong P, Patel R, Sampath R, Ashour AM, Germany LM, et al. "Awake" clipping of cerebral aneurysms: Report of initial series. Journal of Neurosurgery. 2017;**127**:311-318. DOI: 10.3171/2015.12.JNS152140 Erratum in: J Neurosurg. 2017;127:445

[48] Perneczky A, Fries G. Endoscope-assisted brain surgery: Part 1—Evolution, basic concept, and current technique. Neurosurgery. 1998;**42**:219-224; discussion 224

[49] Fischer G, Oertel J, Perneczky A. Endoscopy in aneurysm surgery. Neurosurgery. 2012;**70**:184-190; discussion 190-191. DOI: 10.1227/NEU.0b013e3182376a36

[50] Taniguchi M, Takimoto H, Yoshimine T, Shimada N, Miyao Y, Hirata M, et al. Application of a rigid endoscope to the microsurgical management of 54 cerebral aneurysms: Results in 48 patients. Journal of Neurosurgery. 1999;**91**:231-237

[51] Nishiyama Y, Kinouchi H, Senbokuya N, Kato T, Kanemaru K, Yoshioka H, et al. Endoscopic indocyanine green video angiography in aneurysm surgery: An innovative method for intraoperative assessment of blood flow in vasculature hidden from microscopic view. Journal of Neurosurgery. 2012;**117**:302-308. DOI: 10.3171/2012.5.JNS112300

[52] Andrade-Barazarte H, Patel K, Turel MK, Doglietto F, Agur A, Gentili F, et al. The endoscopic transpterional port approach: Anatomy, technique, and initial clinical experience. Journal of Neurosurgery. 2019;**22**:1-11. DOI: 10.3171/2018.10.JNS171898

[53] Xiao LM, Tang B, Xie SH, Huang GL, Wang ZG, Zeng EM, et al. Endoscopic endonasal clipping of anterior circulation aneurysm: Surgical techniques and results. World Neurosurgery. 2018;**115**:e33-e44. DOI: 10.1016/j.wneu.2018.03.093

[54] Enseñat J, Alobid I, de Notaris M, Sanchez M, Valero R, Prats-Galino A, et al. Endoscopic endonasal clipping of a ruptured vertebral-posterior inferior cerebellar artery aneurysm: Technical case report. Neurosurgery. 2011;**69**:onsE121-onsE127; discussion onsE127-128. DOI: 10.1227/NEU.0b013e318223b637

[55] Khalessi AA, Rahme R, Rennert RC, Borgas P, Steinberg JA, White TG, et al. First-in-man clinical experience using a high-definition 3-dimensional exoscope system for microneurosurgery. Operative Neurosurgery (Hagerstown).

2019;**16**:717-725. DOI: 10.1093/ons/opy320

[56] Langer DJ, White TG, Schulder M, Boockvar JA, Labib M, Lawton MT. Advances in intraoperative optics: A brief review of current exoscope platforms. Operative Neurosurgery (Hagerstown). 2019. pii: opz276. DOI: 10.1093/ons/opz276

[57] Djulejić V, Marinković S, Milić V, Georgievski B, Rašić M, Aksić M, et al. Common features of the cerebral perforating arteries and their clinical significance. Acta Neurochirurgica. 2015;**157**:743-754; discussion 754. DOI: 10.1007/s00701-015-2378-8

[58] Yamamoto Y, Fukuda H, Yamada D, Kurosaki Y, Handa A, Lo B, et al. Association of perforator infarction with clinical courses and outcomes following surgical clipping of ruptured anterior communicating artery aneurysms. World Neurosurgery. 2017;**107**:724-731. DOI: 10.1016/j.wneu.2017.08.086

[59] Zhao M, Charbel FT, Alperin N, Loth F, Clark ME. Improved phase-contrast flow quantification by three-dimensional vessel localization. Magnetic Resonance Imaging. 2000;**18**:697-706

[60] Calderon-Arnulphi M, Amin-Hanjani S, Alaraj A, Zhao M, Du X, Ruland S, et al. In vivo evaluation of quantitative MR angiography in a canine carotid artery stenosis model. AJNR. American Journal of Neuroradiology. 2011;**32**:1552-1559. DOI: 10.3174/ajnr.A2546

[61] Abla AA, Lawton MT. Anterior cerebral artery bypass for complex aneurysms: An experience with intracranial-intracranial reconstruction and review of bypass options. Journal of Neurosurgery. 2014;**120**:1364-1377. DOI: 10.3171/2014.3.JNS132219

[62] van Doormaal TPC, de Boer B, Redegeld S, van Thoor S, Tulleken CAF, van der Zwan A. Preclinical success but clinical failure of the sutureless excimer laser-assisted non-occlusive anastomosis (SELANA) slide. Acta Neurochirurgica. 2018;**160**:2159-2167. DOI: 10.1007/s00701-018-3686-6

Chapter 3

Role of Cranioplasty in Management of Chiari Malformation

Asifur Rahman

Abstract

Chiari malformations (CM) are a set of enigmatic congenital anomalies, owing to their complex pathology, varied presentations and management dilemma. Because of the daunting nature of this disease, a universal definitive treatment protocol is yet to be established. Diverse surgical procedures are in practice with various philosophies, aiming to resolve different sections of the pathologies of this disorder, either singly or in combination. However, outcomes are quite variable. Though not a well-recognized and commonly practiced paradigm of managing CM, different techniques of cranioplasty for CM has been described by many authors with variable rates of success. Cranioplasty for Chiari has been found to be helpful in different circumstances with the objective to address different predicaments. Initially, it has been exercised as one of the modalities to manage some particular situations, mostly in cases to solve complications following surgery. Now in some centers, different types of methods of cranioplasty are practiced routinely to treat particular set of Chiari patients with specifically set criteria and some have shown success in those certain scenarios. In this chapter, different methods of cranioplasty for Chiari malformation by different authors, strategies behind the techniques and their results are described in brief. "Stealth cranioplasty", a technique devised by our team is also portrayed.

Keywords: Chiari malformation, posterior fossa volume, posterior fossa decompression, cranioplasty

1. Introduction

Hans Chiari analytically described his eponymous subset of patients of Chiari malformation (CM) first in 1891. In his subsequent article on CM in 1896, he elaborated the entity and added a new type to his previously described three types. He only described his findings and gave two theories to relate the findings to probable pathogenesis. He thought that the herniation is a result of congenital hydrocephalus, which is a chronic one with early onset that displaces the neural structures through the foramen magnum (FM) into the spinal canal [1]. But that is actually not the case always. The other possibility that he thought of was inadequate bone growth and insufficient enlargement of skull triggering raised intracranial pressure (ICP) leading to force down the hindbrain. Later, with advancements of technologies and further research, Chiari's latter hypothesis appears to be impressively a precise one [1–4]. Some other scientists around that period of Chiari, like Cleland in 1883 and Mennicke in 1891 described about hindbrain herniation and also advocated that the pathology lies in the defective bone around the foramen magnum, which supports the theory of the pathogenesis originating from the small posterior cranial fossa (PCF) [5, 6]. Though, these earlier studies were based on observations of autopsy findings, these theories still are very much contemporary, as verified by the findings of the modern technologies of recent times. However, Chiari or other researchers of his time did not think of solving the problem.

For this puzzling condition, surgery was not contemplated till 1930, when Cornelis Joachimus Van Houweninge Graftdijk, first attempted surgery for CM on a patient with myelomeningocele and ventriculogram-proven hindbrain herniation. He tried to restore better flow of cerebrospinal fluid (CSF) around the craniovertebral junction (CVJ) by widening the space through which the redundant cerebellar tissue had herniated [7]. Since then, attempts to solve the problem of CM by surgery are being practiced and many procedures have been devised and various modifications have been made.

From the very beginning of surgical endeavors, disputes regarding management of CM are a continuing issue of debate because of its intricate and perplexing character. The pathophysiology of syringomyelia (SM) that often exist with CM, seems to be identical and gives the opportunity to solve both with a common procedure, as both CM and SM share the common pathology [8]. The commonest surgical practice for Chiari malformation type 1 (CM1), the commonest of the Chiari malformations, and SM is a simple posterior fossa decompression with the removal of part of posterior arch of C1 combined with variations in the next steps. Reconstruction of the posterior fossa (PF) by cranioplasty is not a routine procedure following posterior fossa decompression (PFD) for the CM1. Many authors described posterior fossa reconstruction with cranioplasty following PFD in many ways with different philosophies. In this chapter, we will discuss the different procedures of cranioplasties performed in surgery for CM1 along with the concepts behind those with elaboration of our thoughts while we do cranioplasty in our technique.

2. Common surgical approaches for Chiari malformation

Development of CM results from developmental anomaly of the occipital bone, rendering the posterior fossa small and shallow, which, along with other factors, leads to herniation of the normal neural elements through the foramen magnum. To reach a unanimous management protocol for CM is challenging owing to the nature of the disorder, its diverse clinical presentations and inexplicable image findings. Depending on presentation in milder forms of symptoms, some authors have advocated conservative management. Nonetheless, surgical intervention remains the gold standard for most of the symptomatic CMs, both in reduction of tonsilar herniation and reestablishment of CSF dynamics around the CVJ; and ultimately in overall outcome. Surgical procedures are many for CM, but no definite single procedure is accepted universally. Keeping the basic techniques identical, many forms and variations are adopted in the procedures and are practiced in different combinations. For many years after Van Houweninge Graftdijk first attempted to treat CM surgically, surgery carried a grave prognosis. At present, with better understanding of the pathology and advances in technology, most patients with CM1 can be benefited by surgical procedures.

The common practice in all surgical approaches is a suboccipital craniectomy with removal of posterior arch of C1. However, there are disagreements and wide range of variations regarding the extent of bone removal and different additional measures taken along with. For management of CM1, dura can be addressed in different ways like leaving the dura intact with removal of the constricting bands only [9], scoring of the dura [10, 11], resection of the outer layer of the dura [12–14], opening the dura and keeping it remain open [15–17], and performing duraplasty with different materials, both natural and artificial [13, 18–24]. The arachnoid manipulation equally differs from leaving it intact by doing an arachnoid preserving durotomy or arachnoid preserving duraplasty [9, 25–27], to opening and resecting it to remove adhesions [8, 19, 23, 28–30]. Dealing the cerebellar tonsils also vary like not touching them [27, 31], separating them by dissection [28, 32], shrinking by bipolar coagulation [13, 19, 23, 33, 34] or carrying out a subpial resection [8, 19, 35, 36]. Recently, minimal invasive endoscopy assisted decompression at the foramen magnum for CM have also been reported [37, 38].

3. An overview of cranioplasties for Chiari malformation

Cranioplasty is not an uncommon procedure in neurosurgery for different conditions. In CM1 surgery, cranioplasty is not a generally prescribed regular technique and thus is not practiced frequently. Most of the times, this is done to manage complications related to routine surgeries for CM1 and sometimes for other types of CM. Whatever the reason is, those who do cranioplasty during CM1 surgery have their own philosophies and the techniques have evolved around the basic pathology of development of CM1 or the complications following regular surgery. Various operative methods for CM and SM have been reported and their efficacy either singly or in combinations in management of CM is still debatable. Most of the authors who practice cranioplasty for the treatment of CM have the theory in their minds that the basic pathology lays in the erroneous architecture of the posterior fossa. Most believe that the posterior fossa is less roomy than the volume of normal neural structures which attributes to herniation of the tonsils through the foramen magnum as well as resulting in disequilibrium of the CSF flow and dynamics between the cranial and the spinal CSF compartments. In some instances, cranioplasty is done routinely in selected cases of CM1. A chronology of cranioplasty procedures for CM with philosophies behind those are portrayed here.

3.1 "Expansive suboccipital cranioplasty" by Tokuno et al.

The very first portrayal of cranioplasty designed for surgery of Chiari malformation found in English literature is by Tokuno et al. in 1987, when they described their technique for treating patients of CM with SM [39]. Till then, the commonest and most popular operative technique of surgery for Chiari was based on the theories of Gardner and William. Tokuno et al. operated on 38 patients over 10 years between 1976 and 1986. A total of 31 out of 38 patients of their series had syringomyelia. In the last 2 years of their study, they carried out an "expansive suboccipital cranioplasty" on their last 17 patients, in addition to Gardner's operation. With the goal of expanding the posterior fossa, they did cranioplasty with autologous suboccipital bone and an iliac bone graft, creating a larger suboccipital bone flap measuring about 5 × 3 × 0.5 cm in size. They followed up all the 38 patients for 1–10 years post-operatively. The addition of "expansive suboccipital cranioplasty" to Gardner's operation resulted in substantially better result in comparison to Gardner's operation alone, with 82% and 67% of good recovery, respectively. Following expansive suboccipital cranioplasty, symptoms of the patients also seemed to improve more rapidly, though a very few patients had transient worsening. By their new operative method, they wanted to obtain a full decompression of the posterior fossa to maintain normal CSF flow around the foramen magnum.

As there was no regular use of MRI for screening or diagnosing CM or SM at that time, they could not measure the volume of the posterior fossa in all of their patients.

However, based on radiological and intra-operative observations of 32% of their patients having narrow posterior fossa, they came to a conclusion that there is disproportion between the suboccipital cavity and the infratentorial content. They also had the premonition that, even if the suboccipital space seems to be normal, the infratentorial component might be relatively too large for that. They devised their procedure with the intention to remodel the neural structures back to a normal physiology by enlarging the posterior fossa through "expansive suboccipital cranioplasty".

3.2 "Expansive suboccipital cranioplasty" by Sakamoto et al.

In 1999, after 12 years of the first report of cranioplasty for Chiari by Tokuno et al., Sakamoto et al. from the same university hospital of Osaka City reported a procedure of cranioplasty for surgery of CM1 associated with SM with some modifications of the procedure of their predecessors. They also termed their technique "expansive suboccipital cranioplasty" (ESC) [40]. Relatively high incidence of postoperative complications and deterioration following the most practiced Gardner's operation, instigated them to devise their technique. During the period between 1985 and 1996, they divided their patients into 2 groups with 20 patients in each group. One group consisted of the patients who underwent ESC together with opening of the foramen of Magendie and plugging of the obex (ESC + PO) from 1985 to 1990 and the other consisted of another 20 patients who underwent ESC but without any intra-arachnoidal procedures between 1991 and 1996.

Their technique of ESC comprised of a large suboccipital osteoplastic craniotomy extending from the FM inferiorly to the margin of the transverse sinus superiorly and 5 cm from the midline laterally on each side along with an osteoplastic laminotomy of the atlas. The FM was enlarged and arachnoid preserving dural opening was carried out ensuring absence of any arachnoid adhesion at the major cistern by intra-operative ultrasound. Duraplasty was done with pericranium. For enlargement of the posterior fossa, the harvested occipital bone flap was fashioned to be expanded by joining the preserved part of the atlas and graft harvested from the outer layer of the cranium at the external protuberance or from the iliac bone. The newly crafted bone flap was then restored and fixed over the craniotomy gap to cover the major cistern. Dural tacking with the bone flap was done to widen the CSF space around the major cistern.

Post-operative MRI revealed enlargement of the major cistern and the whole subarachnoid space of the posterior fossa and reduction of the syrinx size and length in all 40 patients irrespective of clinical improvement. All the 20 patients who underwent ESC, had neurological improvement after surgery without recurrence, while 17 patients improved neurologically and 3 remained unchanged in the ESC + PO group. Based on the theory of a small posterior fossa that may trigger CM and SM, they developed the ESC, targeting to enlarge the small posterior fossa and to obtain a sufficient flow of CSF. They postulated that intra-arachnoid procedures are not necessary to facilitate restoration of CSF flow as by expanding the posterior cranial fossa, the CSF spaces are enlarged and the craniospinal pressure dissociation is also reduced. They also had the impression that the major cistern can be effectively kept open by tacking the dura to the overlying bone flap. They furthermore postulated that ESC can prevent cerebellar slump despite a large craniotomy by avoiding adhesion of the caudal surface of the cerebellum to the dura.

3.3 "Partial suboccipital cranioplasty" by Holly and Batzdorf

Cerebellar ptosis (CP) is not an uncommon occurrence that usually results from too large a craniectomy for CM, which often can potentially refute the desired outcome of the surgery. In 2001, Holly and Batzdorf reported partial suboccipital cranioplasty with or without intradural exploration for cerebellar ptosis following suboccipital craniectomy for CM [41].

Aiming to treat CP following PFD for CM1 effectively, they developed their technique and implemented that on four of the seven symptomatic CP patients. These patients presented with symptoms from 9 months to 17 years following initial surgery. Of the four patients, two patients underwent re-exploration with reduction of the tonsils, pericranial duraplasty and partial suboccipital cranioplasty with hydroxyapatite (HA) in one and with methylmethacrylate (MMA) in the other. Rest of the two patients underwent extradural exploration of the suboccipital craniectomy and partial suboccipital cranioplasty with MMA. All the four patients, who had partial suboccipital cranioplasty with or without intradural exploration produced rewarding results. With their crescent-shaped partial suboccipital cranioplasty the previous 4 × 4 cm suboccipital craniectomies were transformed into approximately 2 × 2 cm ones. To secure the prosthesis, they grooved the contiguous bone edges with high speed drill and injected MMA into the grooves.

Most of these patients of cerebellar sag present with headache and neurological deficits due to persistent obstruction of CSF flow around the CVJ leading to disturbance in CSF flow dynamics. Usually, too large a craniectomy leads to CP, and from that they philosophized that decompression of the posterior fossa extensively is unnecessary to treat a pathology that is primarily around the level of the foramen magnum. They felt that the initial craniectomies were nearly twice as large as necessary and lessened the opening to approximately 2 × 2 cm in all. They basically had the aim to make the posterior fossa as roomy as possible to reestablish the CSF flow dynamics around the FM back to normal without hampering the support for the cerebellum and suggested that enough bone should be left to support the greatest diameter of the cerebellum as a bony supportive shelf. The use of MMA or HA for the cranioplasty was chosen as prosthesis as because these materials can be fixed in place without any additional hardware. Partial suboccipital cranioplasty was successful in treating the headache by supporting the cerebellum and alleviating stretching the dura mater with reversal of the CSF flow obstruction.

3.4 "Supratentorial cranial enlargement" by Di Rocco and Velardi

Chiari malformation is generally a congenital anomaly, but CM can be an acquired event as well. Some literatures in recent time have highlighted the role of the cranio-spinal pressure differential across the foramen magnum in pathogenesis of Acquired Chiari type-1 malformation (ACM1). In 2003, Di Rocco and Velardi drew attention to a different dimension in development of acquired ACM1 in patients that had surgery for raised ICP resulting from causes other than congenital HCP and they treated these patients in their technique [42]. They described two cases of symptomatic ACM1 following lumbo-peritoneal shunt and cystoventriculo-peritoneal shunt for pseudotumor cerebri and suprasellar arachnoid cyst, respectively, in two adolescents. They hypothesized that secondary craniocephalic disproportion plays a substantial role in the genesis of ACM1 in patients having extrathecal CSF shunts.

Both of their patients remained asymptomatic following the initial shunting procedures. However, both became symptomatic after a long interval and MRI revealed ACM1 in both the patients. Di Rocco and Velardi did surgery upon them in their devised technique successfully.

They devised a method of supratentorial cranial decompression by expansive cranioplasty with autologous bone. In their procedure, two parietal bone flaps were made on each side of the sagittal suture. The bone flaps were then raised to augment the supratentorial cranial volume. For sustained elevated position of the bone flaps in order to maintain the enlarged cranial dimension, two small blocks of bone harvested from the posterior parietal margin of the bone flaps were placed between the bone flap and the margin of the craniotomy adjacent to the medial border. Cosmetic aspect of the expanding craniotomy to maintain precise contour of the calvarial surface was meticulously taken care of.

There were marked improvements of the symptoms of both the patients. Headache and papilledema in the first patient and diplopia, papilledema, retinal hemorrhage, headache, mild right hemiparesis and mild dysmetria of the left upper limb in the second patient—all subsided. Post-operative MRI showed significant regression of tonsillar caudal descent in both the patients.

Pathogenesis of ACM1 is most likely multifactorial and its development following extrathecal shunts can be explained by the "craniospinal pressure gradient" theory and the "cephalocranial disproportion" theory. They theorized from their observations that placement of the extrathecal shunt in children leads to cessation of cranial growth as well as results in progressive thickening of the cranial vault by inner apposition of bone, which spans for years. Further observation of upward displacement of the upper cerebellar vermis to lodge upward into the quadrigeminal cistern along with the caudal herniation of the cerebellar tonsils, firmly establishes the fact of overcrowding of the neural structures within the posterior cranial fossa. When cephalocranial disproportion is the main factor responsible for ACM1 in these cases, it was logical for them to go for the cranial expansion as a whole to create more supratentorial intracranial space by autologous bone cranioplasty to dismiss the cephalocranial disproportion, which yielded satisfactory result. This alleviated the need for manipulation of the shunts as well.

3.5 "One-stage posterior decompression and fusion" by Nishikwawa et al.

In 2004, Nishikwawa et al. came with their method of one stage expansive cranioplasty with autologous bone and rigid occipitocervical fixation for CM1 associated with various degrees of other anomalies in two patients [43]. Their patients presented with various symptoms like occipitalgia, chest pain and numbness from face to both hands. Radiologically, there were occipitalization of the atlas, mild form of AAD, ventral compression of the cervicomedullary junction by the basilar invagination, Chiari malformation and syringomyelia Additionally, the second patient had possible slump of the cerebellum following foramen magnum decompression with small craniectomy and splitting the dura elsewhere 12 years previously.

A large suboccipital osteoplastic craniotomy in the first case and extension of the previous suboccipital craniectomy in the second case was performed. Ultasonographic confirmation of pulsation of the tonsils was done to ensure adequate decompression. Safety of the screw insertion was verified from preoperative and peroperative simulation by computerized navigation system for two cervical transarticular screws through the lateral mass of the axis into the lateral mass of the occipitalized atlas in patient 1 and into the pedicle of the axis in patient 2. Guide holes along the diploic space on the margin of the craniotomy in the 1st patient and oblique burr hole at the margin of the craniotomy on each side in the 2nd patient were made. Rigid occipitoaxial fixation was accomplished by connecting the diploic screws to the pedicle or transarticular screws with a rod on each side. The autologous bone flap was secured with titanium wires. Finally, dural tacking sutures connecting the dura to the overlying bone were done.

Both the patients had remarkable recovery of their symptoms with notable expansion of the posterior fossa with an enlarged CSF space in MRI and good fusion of the grafted bones in 3D CT scan. They innovated the technique of simultaneous occipitocervical fusion in addition to their regularly practiced method of posterior fossa decompression and expansive cranioplasty for implantation of screw in the occipital diploic space for stabilization and fusion of occipitocervical instability in Chiari patients with syrinx, basilar invagination and AAD. They opined that diploic screws can be used safely for occipital fixation irrespective of the size of the suboccipital craniectomy and in cases of mobile and partially or completely reducible atlantoaxial dislocation. However, a synchronized stabilization in the optimally reduced position is mandatory for successful fusion.

3.6 "Simple technique for expansive suboccipital cranioplasty" by Takayasu et al.

Takayasu et al. made posterior fossa reconstruction simpler and easier by autologous cranioplasty for CM with SM and described this procedure on 14 patients in 2001 and on 16 patients in 2004 [44, 45]. The basic idea of this method was also to expand the volume of the PCF, thus they too call it expansive suboccipital cranioplasty like their preceding Japanese colleagues. They performed their procedures on patients of syringomyelia associated with Chiari I malformation since 1992. Different symptoms and signs in their patients included sensory disturbances, motor weakness, brainstem and/or cerebellar signs and intractable pain.

In their simpler procedure, they first did an en bloc upper suboccipital craniotomy, keeping the foramen magnum margin intact. Under the microscope with the help of air drill, Kerrison punches and rongeurs, the posterior bony margin of the FM is removed. The C1 posterior arch is removed to the maximum along with the upper part of the C2 lamina if the tonsils extended beyond C2. Arachnoid preserving duraplasty with fascia lata was done. The thick internal crista of the occipital bone flap is removed and the flap is shaped to fit the lower portion of the craniectomy gap to cover the FM. Expansive cranioplasty is accomplished by fixing the tailored bone flap with titanium miniplates. In some cases, the flap was replaced inside-out to buy more space and to have a better fit. Tacking of the dural graft with the bone graft and packing of bone chips into the upper craniectomy defect, reinforced with fibrin glue, was done to complete the cranioplasty.

All the patients improved clinically significantly within a few weeks of surgery, except 2. Both had persistent dysesthetic pain, one of whom improved within several months. In follow-up of more than 1 year most of the patients showed marked improvement in terms of ascent of tonsils and resolution of size of syringes.

They did the cranioplasty with the intension to prevent complications like pseudomeningocele and CSF leakage by providing support for the dural closure. Furthermore, posterior fossa reconstruction has the potential to prevent relapse of symptoms from restenosis of the cisterna magna, cerebellar ptosis and wound depression. Their method is simpler than the others as this only needs repositioning of the bone flap on the bony defect.

3.7 "Cranioplasty using hydroxyapatite implants" by Itoh et al.

Itoh et al. described a procedure of cranioplasty with a curved plate of Hydroxyapatite for Treatment of Syringomyelia associated with Chiari I Malformation, in 2001 [46]. They applied their method on eight patients diagnosed on basis of clinical examinations and neuroradiological findings of MRI and 3D-CT over a period of 19 months. All patients had varying degrees of sensory discomfort of the extremities with the mean duration of symptoms for 40 months. The most frequent complaint was unilateral dysesthesia in the upper extremity. MRI revealed tonsillar herniation and syrinx of various degrees and extents. Phase-contrast cine-MRI displayed absence of CSF flow in the retrotonsillar subarachnoid space and to-and-fro drift within the syrinx.

In their technique, they first did foramen magnum decompression by a suboccipital craniectomy as in other procedures along with C1 laminectomy in seven cases and did C1 and C2 upper dome laminectomies in one case. In three cases, they did duraplasty with Gore-Tex membrane and resected the outer layer of the dura in five cases. Cranioplasty to cover the craniectomy gap as well as to expand the posterior fossa was performed using HA implants in all cases. They did tenting of the dura or the duraplasty with the implants in all cases.

In a mean follow-up period of 13.3-months, five patients improved and three patients remained unchanged. Postoperative syrinx resolution was seen in seven patients on MRI. HA cranioplasty had to be removed in one patient because of development of an epidural abscess, but this patient had no further neurological deterioration. Six months after surgery, 3D-CT revealed the HA implant to be integrated with the adjacent occipital bone. They used HA, as a substitute for autologous bone grafts, for expansive cranioplasty to enlarge small posterior fossa to establish better CSF flow at the major cistern. The use of HA was to reduce the chance of absorption of the autologous bone in the long run if used for cranioplasty. Moreover, it is technically easy to use the HA implants. The idea of tenting the dura with the cranioplasty was to inhibit the retention of CSF at epidural space following surgery.

3.8 "Simple and safe method of cranial reconstruction" by Sheikh et al.

In 2006, Sheikh et al. described a simple method of cranioplasty that they applied for posterior fossa reconstruction for many procedures including Chiari malformation [47]. They depicted their easy modified procedure of cranioplasty utilizing patient's own bone dust, tissue glue and gel foam sheets. Ten patients underwent posterior fossa reconstruction between the period of 2000 and 2004 for different pathologies including CM.

After exposure of the suboccipital bone, craniectomy is done by doing multiple burr holes and connecting them with a high-speed drill. Produced bone dust is meticulously collected, preserved and kept wet in a container with small amount of antibiotic treated saline. Following craniectomy and water tight dural closure, a layer of tissue glue is applied over the dura. Two sheets of gel foam are fashioned to fit the craniectomy defect. The bone dust is dried to make dough and is spread between the 2 layers of the gel foam sheets and is held together with tissue glue. The bone dust sandwich is placed over the craniectomy defect separated from the overlying muscle layer by another sheet of gel foam to complete the cranioplasty.

Post-operative plain and 3D CT scan in follow-up of 11–36 months showed excellent reconstruction of the posterior fossa bony contour with the cranioplasty. Two patients needed redo surgery after 6 weeks of cranioplasty which revealed interesting findings. In both the patients, the cranioplasty was totally separated from the suboccipital musculature and the dura. No other complication was noted.

They devised this quick and safe reconstruction technique to prevent the persistent post craniectomy headache due to dural stretching from musculo-fibrous adhesion with the dura as well as to give a better cosmetic result by preventing depression at the craniectomy site. Their procedure of making a bone dust sandwich was better than putting the bone dust directly on the craniectomy gap as the dust is not dispersed. The gel foam used for the cranioplasty also hold some blood which help in ingrowth of osteoblasts to form new bone. This simple and easy procedure had a satisfactory and effective result both clinically and radiologically.

3.9 "Posterior cranial fossa box expansion" by Heller et al.

Heller et al. portrayed a new method of "posterior cranial fossa box expansion" for MRI confirmed symptomatic cerebellar ptosis following cranial vault decompression for Chiari I malformations in 2007 [48]. They operated on seven patients, who had undergone posterior fossa decompression for CM and developed symptomatic cerebellar ptosis for 12 ± 1 months from the initial surgery at other institutions. Their patients presented with headache, upper extremity numbness, paresthesia, respiratory disturbance and walking difficulty from cerebellar ptosis.

Through the previous incision, the previous suboccipital craniectomy was delineated. In the next steps of the procedure, a split thickness square calvarial bone graft, approximately 2–3 cm larger than the width of foramen magnum is harvested from the occipital bone, just below the lambdoid suture. With the help of reciprocating saw and bone cutter, the bone graft is fashioned for the box reconstruction by trisecting the approximately 1 cm wide upper and lower margins into equal 3 segments which leaves six split-thickness pieces and one large rectangular graft. The smaller grafts are stacked into three stacks of two grafts each and fixed with screw at the upper and the two lateral margins of the foramen magnum in an inverted "U" manner. The rectangular bone graft is placed and fixed with the three legs of the bone graft stacks to create a concave dome of bone over the foramen magnum. The box cranioplasty is then completed to cover the cerebellum, separating the surrounding soft tissues and reducing the foramen magnum defect significantly.

All their patients were symptom free in a follow-up period of more than 12 months and resolution of cerebellar ptosis in all seven patients and collapse of syrinx in five of the seven patients were confirmed by MRI.

They felt that the cerebellar ptosis is a combination of lack of mechanical support from PFD and pressure-dissociation of CSF causing a sucking effect. As they acknowledged the need of cerebellar support, with their procedure they reduced previous craniectomy gap around the foramen magnum to 2 × 3 cm from over 4 × 4 cm. As a whole their box reconstruction cranioplasty resulted in expansion of the posterior cranial fossa with support to prevent cerebellar ptosis and preservation of pressure dissociation equilibrium around the cisterna magna with the added benefit of maintenance of separation between the neck musculature and soft tissues from the neural tissue. They infer that posterior fossa box reconstruction can resolve symptomatology of cerebellar sag without any intradural manipulation.

3.10 "Partial suboccipital cranioplasty" by Di et al.

Di et al. described cranioplasty related to surgery for CM in 2008 [49]. They reported about critical complication of respiratory arrest in 2 patients following partial cranioplasty for cerebellar ptosis subsequent to PFD for CM. One patient developed symptoms like recurrent and intractable headache and gait disturbance for 1 year following surgery for CM 2 years previously, while the other had developed mild headache, dizziness, difficulty in swallowing, gait imbalance, progressive numbness in the face and upper extremities and occasional urinary incontinence for 4 years following PFD 7 years back. Both the patients had severe cerebellar ptosis on MRI.

Both the patients underwent a partial suboccipital cranioplasty. Per-operatively large suboccipital craniectomy gaps were identified in both where the cerebellar hemispheres protruded out of the previous craniectomy gap. Only duraplasty was done in one while tonsillar cautery and duraplasty was done in the other. Partial suboccipital cranioplasty with titanium mesh and MMA in one and only with MMA in other was accomplished to reduce the previous craniectomy gap to approximately 2 × 2 cm in size.

Both the patients suffered from similar episodes of apnea and subsequent respiratory arrest, 15 h and 72 h post-operatively, respectively. No bleeding, infarct and blockage of the CSF pathway was seen in the post-operative MRI or CT scan. Chest radiographs were also normal. Both were reintubated and monitored in an intensive care unit. One of them was extubated within 24 h and was discharged home 1 week after, while, extubation failed twice in the other and recovery to a near independent state was achieved after a prolonged mechanical ventilation, with tracheostomy.

Among various post-operative complications, cerebellar ptosis, which usually results from a large craniectomy, has a potentially severe consequence, and its incidence is possibly underestimated. Partial suboccipital cranioplasty has been used to treat the cerebellar ptosis to minimize the large craniectomy gap and to support the cerebellum. The respiratory arrest in these patients is thought to be from stretching on the vulnerable and damaged brainstem by the elevation of the cerebellum during the cerebellar shelving process. There might have been some compromised vasculature too, which surely could play a role.

3.11 "Autologous cranioplasty" by Chou et al.

In 2009, Chou et al. published a technical note on a cranioplasty technique that they devised for treatment for CM [50]. They believed that adherence between muscle and dura, together with the development of occipital neuromas, are the factors of common postoperative complaint of headache. They made some modifications to the conventional craniectomy with the aim to expansion of the posterior fossa. They performed suboccipital craniotomy in their technique on six patients with CM1.

They performed a rectangular craniotomy extending from just below the nuchal line down to the foramen magnum. Following duraplasty, with the help of a Leibinger plate attached to the inner table, the craniotomy flap was fixed to the outer table of the skull with 2 mm screws to elevate the bone flap and to expand the posterior fossa volume as well.

They followed-up the patients for 7 months on average. Post-operative headaches in all the patients improved within 3–4 weeks and there had been no complication. Patients with syringomyelia had complete resolution of syringes. Improvement was seen in overall quality of life of the patients. Three-dimensional analysis of posterior fossa volume revealed effective increase in posterior fossa volume on average, from pre-operative 168 cc to post-operative 192 cc.

Small and shallow posterior fossa is recognized to be the prime factor in development of CM. The authors felt the need of the posterior fossa to be expanded. Consequently, they devised their technique of decompression and expansion of the posterior fossa. With their procedure they also eliminated the possibility of fibrous adhesion between nuchal musculature and the exposed dura to reduce the chance of post-operative headache and neckache during motion from dural stretching. Cranioplasty with autologous bone has the added advantage of reducing local tissue reaction and edema by artificial grafts.

3.12 "Cranioplasty" by Furtado et al.

Furtado et al. reported the management of rare entity of Chiari 3 malformation (CM3) by cranioplasty among other measures in 2009 [51]. Their patient, a 15 months old girl was presented with titubation and occipito-cervical encephalocele since birth. She also had downbeat nystigmus. MRI revealed an occipito-cervical encephalocele containing cerebellum, brainstem and both the occipital poles, in a shallow posterior fossa. 3D CT scan showed a big gap in the occipital bone with mal-development of the C1 and C2 posterior arches.

On surgery, after excising the gliotic cerebellum and the occipital lobes, a meticulous watertight dural closure was accomplished. The large bony gap in the occipital bone was covered with a 5 × 5 cm methylmethacrylate cranioplasty that was fixed with the margin of the occipital bone with steel wire. The remaining occipital lobe, transverse sinus and the upper part of the cerebellum were well contained within the cranioplasty. Wound was covered with an occipital rotation skin flap.

Recovery was uneventful and the baby was discharged home after 5 days. Her lower cranial nerves were intact and there was no HCP. Follow-up CT scan at 3 year showed no bone growth along the cranioplasty margin and she had retarded physical and mental development.

They introduced a variant of cranioplasty procedure to cover and support the transverse sinus and the occipital lobe in a case of CM3. They did cranioplasty with the goal to prevent further herniation of the remaining cerebellar tissue by reducing the gap down to half. Though the functional outcome of CM3 is grave most of the times, surgery is recommended.

3.13 "Expansile suboccipital cranioplasty" by Oro et al.

Oro et al. in 2011 reported the largest series of expansile cranioplasty for CM1 [52]. They described their technique that they applied on 241 patients of fresh Chiari malformation or on recurrent CM patients.

In 2004, they developed a preformed crescent shaped titanium plate to treat CM1 patients by expansile suboccipital cranioplasty. Their titanium plate was designed to cover a craniectomy defect measuring 3 cm wide. Larger crescent plates that can cover 4 cm craniectomies also exist and plates to cover wider decompressions for post-surgical patients can also be customized. Besides, they developed a triangular plate for smaller triangular-shaped craniectomies. After the desired craniectomy, once the suitable plate is selected, it is manually bent into a curved arch and fixed to cover the upper two-thirds to three-fourths of the craniectomy with five to six small screws. No plate dislodgements have been detected in follow-up MRI. The use of the plate is straightforward and they are redesigning the plate to provide more coverage.

The goals of surgery are to achieve dorsal and dorsolateral decompression with restoration of normal CSF dynamics at the CVJ and reduction of the surgical risks.

The expected extent of craniectomy, which varies from 2.7 to 3 cm and the size of the duraplasty, approximately 1.5–2 cm less than the base length, are planned from the T2 sagittal MRI of the CVJ. Planning for inclusion of a C1 laminectomy, and on rare occasions a partial C2 laminectomy, depends on the extent of tonsillar herniation, and the degree of tonsillar and brainstem compression.

They designed their cranioplasty with the goal to provide a rigid surface for attachment of the suboccipital muscles to prevent formation of scar to dura. This process can also prevent "soft spot" headache and reduce the possibility of injury to the area.

3.14 "Cranioplasty with titanium plate" by Rekate and Bristol

In 2012, Rekate and Bristol described their method of cranioplasty following foramen magnum decompression for CM1 [53]. They only described their procedure, but did not provide any patient data. They applied their technique both in adults and in children.

In their method, the rim of the foramen magnum is removed to a distance of 1.5–2.0 cm. The posterior arch of C1 and the laminae and spinous process of C2, when felt necessary, are removed along with the ligamentum flavum. Dura is opened in a linear fashion starting from the spinal dura and then extending upwards upto the bone margin. The fourth ventricle is entered into, to see and lyse the veil, which the authors claim to be typically present and advocates that the veil must be opened to visualize the porcelain white floor of the fourth ventricle. Duraplasty is performed with pericranium, which is sewn in place with absorbable or nonabsorbable suture. Cranioplasty is done with a titanium plate that has been developed only to extend over the craniectomy gap around the foramen magnum and fixed with screws on both sides. The preformed plate allows for custom fitting depending on the patient's anatomy and the extent of the bony opening. A tenting is taken from the center of the graft to the titanium plate.

They set their goals of surgery to remove the compression from the brainstem and reestablish normal CSF dynamics at the CVJ. The dura was opened and the arachnoid around the tonsils was dissected to see the floor of the fourth ventricle with the theory in mind that this maneuver does not add morbidity to the procedure. The aim of dural closure with a patch graft is to create a larger CSF space around the CVJ. The cranioplasty is done mainly to prevent the scarring of the graft to the underlying tonsils.

3.15 "Expansile suboccipital cranioplasty with titanium mesh-assisted dural tenting" by Assina

Assina et al. in 2014 described their process of titanium mesh-assisted dural tenting and expansile suboccipital cranioplasty for preventing cerebellar ptosis following posterior fossa decompression for CM1 [54]. Cerebellar ptosis and dural prolapse or collapse of the cisterna magna are well-recognized complications following PFD. Almost one-third of the operated patients come back with recurrence in their lifetime, often from ptosis and dural prolapse.

They developed their method to prevent cerebellar ptosis and dural prolapse by the technique of titanium mesh-assisted dural tenting and expansile suboccipital cranioplasty. They performed surgery by this procedure on four patients of CM1, three of whom had associated syrinx. All presented with suboccipital headache.

Their craniectomy was extended to the posterior aspect of the occipital condyles laterally. A partial laminectomy of the C2 was done sometimes when the tonsils were extended down to C2. Arachnoid preserving dural opening was performed in a "Y"-shaped fashion superiorly and upside down "T" fashion inferiorly to have a larger dural opening. After watertight duraplasty, a titanium mesh cranioplasty, covering the superior aspect of the craniectomy was done and 2-3 dural tentings were tied with the cranioplasty.

All the patients had uneventful post-operative course without any complication in mean follow-up period of 19 months. In follow-up MRI at 1 year no cerebellar ptosis, collapse or restenosis of cisterna magna, obstruction of CSF pathway requiring re-do surgery was evident. All the patients had improvement of their symptoms and radiographic resolution of syrinx. By this expansile titanium mesh cranioplasty, in addition to expanding the volume of the posterior fossa, they also had the aim to prevent the cerebellar sag by the support of the cranioplast and dural prolapse and the collapse of the cisterna magna by the dural tenting with the cranioplasty. The titanium mesh also has the extra preventive accomplishment against re-stenosis at the CVJ by creating a barrier between the musculature and the dura.

3.16 "Modified pi-technique of reduction cranioplasty" by Choi et al.

Choi et al. in 2014 described reduction cranioplasty in an infant of congenital HCP, occipital encephalocele with CM1 [55]. Though it was not a conventional posterior fossa decompression surgery the presence of CM1 carries the merit to be mentioned here.

They reported a baby of occipital encephalocele diagnosed antenatally by USG. MRI at the age of 1 day revealed severe hydrocephalus, occipital encephalocele and herniation of the lower brainstem and cerebellum into the cervical defect. The baby underwent multiple surgeries from the age of day 1, like repair of the encephalocele, VP shunt, foramen magnum decompression, ETV and EVD for multiple times. Despite all these measures, macrocephaly persisted and anterior fontanelle was open and bulged at 32 months postnatally.

The cranial vault was reshaped by modified pi-procedure of reduction cranioplasty. The gap at the anterior fontanalle was covered with two paired sagittal-parietal bone flaps and the coronal bone flap was advanced to the midline to cover the bone defect. To allow the brain to expand laterally, multiple barrel stave osteotomy was done at the level of the squamosal suture bilaterally.

Postoperatively, the skull defect at the non-fused fontanelle was closed. The skull vault circumference decreased from 58 to 53 cm and correction of macrocephally was seen. There were no postoperative complications. However, they did not mention about the post-operative status of the CM1. Early in infancy, the patient had considerable developmental delays in early infancy. Nevertheless, slow neurological improvement was witnessed during the overall course of development of the baby.

The Chiari malformations are a complex of hindbrain deformities associated hydrocephalus in a minority of patients that need to be managed during the initial stages, which can be cumbersome. Different CSF diversion procedures, even with multiple attempts can lead to craniocerebral disproportion due to discrepancy between the volume of the brain and the volume of the cranium. They recommended that patients of CM1 with other congenital anomalies and HCP can be satisfactorily managed by reduction cranioplasty utilizing the modified pi-technique.

3.17 "Posterior fossa reconstruction using titanium plate" by Udani et al.

In 2014, Udani et al. described their technique of partial posterior fossa cranioplasty using perforated titanium plate for treating cerebellar ptosis and dural ectasia following posterior fossa decompression [56].

They described 12 patients, who previously had undergone PFD for CM1. The interval ranged from 2 to 12 years between the initial surgery and the cranioplasty. First surgery consisted of different combinations of procedures like durapasty, tonsillar shrinkage or syrinx shunting in addition to PFD. Patients presented with headache, neck and back pain, gait ataxia, limb weakness, sensory changes and nystagmus. Imaging revealed persistent tonsillar descent. Four patients had bulging dural ectasia and eight patients had ptosis. Three of the patients had recurrent syrinx.

Five patients, including the three with syrinx, had a 1- to 2-week trial of suboccipital counter pressure with a soft foam rubber pad against the decompression site that was held in place with an elastic bandage, prior to partial titanium cranioplasty and had symptomatic improvement with this trial. Prior craniectomy defects were defined in all the patients per-operatively. A suboccipital perforated titanium plate was shaped to make it slightly convex in the midline and flat on the sides to merge with the bone. It was placed along the inferior edge of the craniectomy to support the dura over the cerebellar hemispheres but not extending down to the foramen magnum and was fixed with the bone using four 4-mm mini screws. Seven patients had intradural exploration with duraplasty with a composite dural graft.

In the mean follow-up period of 18 months, symptoms of four patients with dural ectasia improved significantly. Syrinx improved in two of the three patients. Overall, 10 out of 12 patients responded favorably to the partial titanium cranioplasty.

The cerebellar ptosis, which may develop as a delayed and potentially serious complication, has the potential to reestablish contact with the brainstem, recreating partial obstruction of CSF flow. This in turn may re-establish conditions for filling of a syrinx cavity which is usually a consequence of large craniectomies. They theorized that larger craniectomies are not necessary to accomplish tonsillar decompression.

3.18 "Hemicranioplasty for osteopetrosis and CM1" by Alsahlawi et al.

Alsahlawi et al. reported a case of autosomal-dominant type of osteopetrosis with concomitant CM1, who had headache and severe visual deterioration, all attributing to increased ICP [57]. Osteopetrosis, a disease of abnormal bone density and volume, resulting from imbalance between osteoblastic formation and osteoclastic resorption, usually presents to a neurosurgeon with features of raised ICP. However, association of osteopetrosis and Chiari malformation is rare.

Their patient presented with gradual deteriorating vision, generalized pain in back, limbs and face, and occasional dizziness and tinnitus. Bone mineral density was high and CT scan revealed generalized diffuse thickening of the skull vault and secondary narrowing of the skull base foramina and internal acoustic meatus. MRI demonstrated crowding at the foramen magnum with bilateral cerebellar tonsillar herniation. There was also severe bilateral compression of the cerebral hemispheres with effacement of the ventricles and the subarachnoid spaces. Medical treatment and left sided optic nerve fenestration failed to resolve the symptoms, rather the patient continued to deteriorate and elective hemicranioplasty was performed after 6 weeks of fenestration.

A right sided fronto-pareital craniotomy flap, measuring 14 × 12 cm, was made with the help of 6 burr holes connected by making grooves with drill first and then with craniotome to cover the thickness of the bone. The inner table of the craniotomy flap was thinned out with saw and drill to reduce the thickness from 30 to 8 mm. The brain under pressure was relieved by duraplasty. Cranioplasty was done with the thinned bone with help of mesh and micro plates. Their plan was to do bilateral decompression, but brain was found to be relaxed after performing the procedure on right side.

Immediately after surgery, the patient noticed significant relief of headache. At 6-month follow-up, headache had resolved completely and vision improved markedly. Postop CT scan showed relief of the brain compression evidenced by enlargement of the ventricles and the subarachnoid spaces. Marked improvement of the cerebellar tonsillar herniation was also observed.

Presently, there exists no medical cure for osteopetrosis. Neurosurgical management evolve around symptom relief mainly. Because of severe headache and progressive visual loss, the authors decided to be aggressive in approach. In absence of osteoclastic activity, thickening of the bones led to raised ICP as well as smaller posterior fossa which ultimately resulted in herniation of the tonsils and following decompressive hemicranioplasty, both the raised ICP and tonsillar herniation were markedly relieved.

3.19 "Expansive suboccipital cranioplasty" by Korshunov

Korshunov et al. described their method of expansive suboccipital cranioplasty for CM1 in 2017 [58]. Their patient presented with intensive disabling persistent headache and cervico-occipital pain. The patient also had two attacks of generalized tonic seizures with loss of consciousness. Neurological examination revealed horizontal nystagmus. MRI revealed wedge-shaped tonsillar herniation down to 17 mm below the foramen magnum. There was no HCP or syrinx.

The thickened and deformed margin of the foramen magnum was widely dissected following a posterior fossa midline osteoplastic craniotomy. Posterior arch of the atlas was also resected. Arachnoid preserving duraplasty was performed with collagen matrix patch graft. The thickness of the free bone flap was reduced by grinding and the margin of the foramen magnum on the bone flap was also widened. The upper edge of the bone flap was fixed at the upper margin of the craniectomy defect by silk sutures. The lower part of the flap was pulled outwards and fixed with two resorbable mini-plates to create new space in the lower portion of the PCF.

Immediate postop CT scan revealed satisfactory cranioplasty. At 3 months follow-up, the patient was totally free of headache, cervico-occipital pain and seizure and MRI revealed resolution of tonsillar herniation and reformation of the occipital cistern.

Posterior decompression of the craniovertebral junction is the most common treatment for CM1. In addition to the conventional procedure, the authors tried to expand the posterior fossa with the aim to normalize CSF circulation at the CVJ with some modification. The whole procedure renders a better dural closure with less chance of complications, less chance of compression from inside and outside because of the bony barrier and better chance of reformation of the occipital cistern.

3.20 "Upside down-inside out cranioplasty" by Tjokorda and Tjokorda

Tjokorda and Tjokorda described a method of a less invasive suboccipital decompression-cranioplasty in 2018 [59]. They analyzed retrospectively, 10 patients from 2010 to 2016, on whom they performed their formulated method of upside down-inside out (UDIO) cranioplasty.

Seven patients in their 4th decade or older and three patients in their 3rd decade or younger had Chiari malformation type I with or without syringomyelia.

With the help of pneumatic perforator and drill, a reverse triangular-shaped craniotomy was done in one piece. Laminectomy of C1 and duraplasty was performed, ensuring normal cerebrospinal fluid flow and dural pulsation. The triangular bone flap harvested from the suboccipital craniotomy was replaced upside down-inside out and was fixed with titanium mini plate and screws.

All patients had improvement of their sensory and motor functions immediately following surgery. Post-operative Japanese Orthopedic Association scoring system (JOA score) scores compared to pre-operative scores were improved in all the patients. Only one patient needed a syringo-subarachnoid shunt for syrinx. No acute or late surgical complications were encountered in a follow-up period of at least 12 months.

The philosophy behind putting the bone upside down and inside out was to place the bone graft above the external table of its origin with periosteum inside to increase the posterior fossa volume, prevent re-stenosis and dural scarring. Other benefits of UDIO were thought to be protecting the cerebellum from adhesion or sagging, and this was believed to prevent adhesion, preventing formation of the pseudomeningocele, facilitating the reconstruction of the posterior neck muscles and preventing CSF leak by reducing the suction effect.

3.21 "Cranial vault remodeling" by Valentini et al.

In 2019, Valentini et al. described cranial vault remodeling of five children in a special subset of CM1 with untreated sagittal stenosis (USS) [60]. Association of

CM1 with craniosynostosis is not uncommon and coexistent low cranial volume, especially the small posterior fossa with venous engorgement and hydrocephalus has the potential to contribute in developing symptomatic CM1 in infants.

From a series of 636 CM1 children, from 1998 to 2018, 48 cases of untreated sagittal synostosis associated with CM1 were analyzed. Of the 48 children, 27 children were operated for different signs and symptoms like headache, intellectual disability, behavioral disorders, visual loss, sleep apneas, raised ICP, papilledema, syringomyelia and scoliosis. Different modalities of surgical procedures were performed and 5 of the children underwent cranial vault remodeling. Three of them had only cranial vault remodeling, while craniovertebral decompression (CVD) was also performed on 1 before and on 1 after the remodeling.

They did a complete cranial vault remodeling, by means of a personal free flaps technique, adopting the osteo-distraction techniques used for complex craniosynostosis. The flaps were extended on the sagittal area also to favor vertical and wide enlargement.

All the patients had improved symptomatically. In postop MRI they had restoration of normal posterior fossa CSF flow with tonsillar ascent or stabilization, and shrinkage or control of the syrinx diameter.

This procedure was aimed to increase the skull volume, both supra and infratentorial, to reduce the struggle for space between cerebrum and cerebellum. The pathogenesis of CM1 in sagittal stenosis (SS) has been explained by the downward compensatory cranial growth. USS causes a constraint to the posterior cranial vault vertical expansion, resulting in a posterior fossa smaller than normal. The reduced supratentorial volume contributes to downward cerebellar migration directly or through the increase of ICP, and probably also related to the venous hypertension due to superior sagittal sinus constriction in the bony groove. They suggested that the double causal factor in SS, the competition for volume between cerebrum and cerebellum; and the small posterior fossa, both need a surgical intervention by cranial vault remodeling and by CVD respectively. The observations suggest, SS carries the risk to develop a symptomatic CM1, when left untreated, is not amenable by CVD alone.

3.22 "Stealth cranioplasty" by Rahman et al.: our technique and thoughts

In 2017, we described a novel technique of reconstruction of posterior fossa by cranioplasty with the use of pre-shaped titanium mesh for CM1, which we call "Stealth cranioplasty" [27]. In the procedure, we set our goal to address all possible symptoms with maintenance of the surgical modifications continually as well as to prevent complications and recurrence.

We performed surgery in our method on 11 adult patients of CM1 with SM, who presented between 2012 and early 2017. Neurological symptoms of the patients included sensory disturbance, neckache, limb weakness and suboccipital headache for a duration of 6–84 months. MRI of all the patients demonstrated cerebellar tonsillar descent more than 5 mm from the foramen magnum and syringes of different diameters, extending from 3 to more than 10 levels.

A midline posterior fossa craniectomy measuring about 3 × 2.5 cm and laminectomy of the C1 posterior arch about 1 cm on both sides from the midline is done (**Figure 1A**). An arachnoid preserving midline linear durotomy (**Figure 1B**) followed by duraplasty with a patch of investing layer of the deep cervical fascia is performed (**Figure 1C**). Six tacking sutures are taken from the cut margins of the dura; 2 on both sides and 1 each from the upper and lower tips of the opening (**Figure 1B** and **C**).

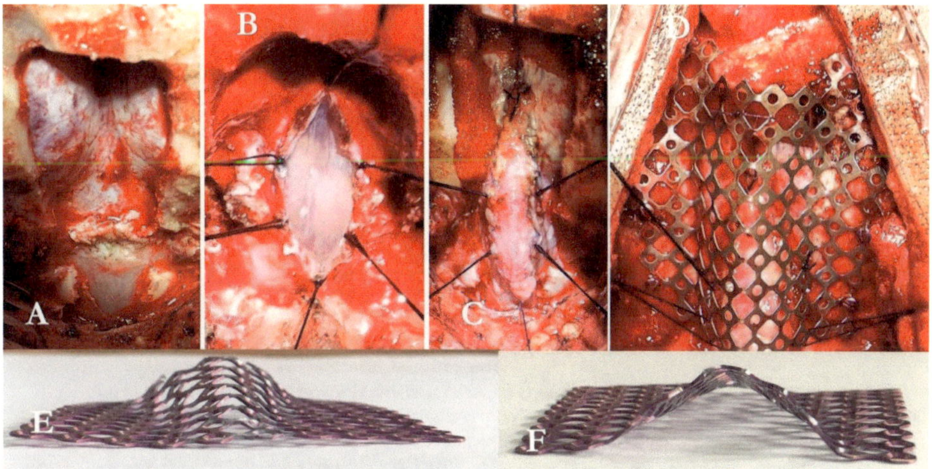

Figure 1.
Different stages of stealth cranioplasty: (A) craniectomy and C1 posterior arch laminectomy, (B) arachnoid preserving durotomy and 6 tackings from the margin, (C) duraplasty, (D) placing of the stealth cranioplast and tenting, (E) stealth cranioplast from front and (F) from rear.

A titanium mesh measuring about 5 × 5 cm is bent in the middle into a longitudinally half split cone to mimic the cockpit and the flat sides of the mesh are bent outwards to give them the contour of the wings of a Stealth bomber (**Figure 1E** and **F**). The widened part of the cone is cut in a crescent to create more space around the CVJ. The titanium mesh Stealth cranioplast is placed over the craniectomy gap with the wider portion at the lower end over the foramen magnum and is fixed with 6–7 mini screws. The six tackings are now tacked with the cranioplasty giving the duraplasty the shape of a hexagonal tent (**Figure 1D**).

The "stealth cranioplasty" augments the posterior fossa volume and maintains that and the tacking of the duraplasty maintains the patency of the newly formed cisterna magna.

All the patients of the series were followed up for a period of 7–54 months. Eight patients improved having a Chicago Chiari Outcome Scale (CCOS) score of 13–15, while 3 patients remained unchanged. All the patients had remarkable shape change of the posterior fossa from a flat lower part to a spherical and voluminous lower part on postop CT scan. Diameter of the FM also increased evidently (**Figure 2A** and **B**). On post-operative MRI, good re-establishment of cisterna magna was noted in all the patients. Marked reduction of syrinx was observed in two patients (**Figure 2C** and **D**). Eight patients had moderate to mild reduction of syrinx while one patient had no change. No post-operative complication or worsening of pre-operative symptoms were seen and none of the patients needed redo surgery.

Though our technique is not an all-encompassing one, we developed our novel procedure based on the well-established theory of overcrowded shallow posterior fossa causing herniation of the contents through the foramen magnum. We thought of cranioplasty first to make more space in the posterior fossa, especially around the foramen magnum as well as to prevent recurrence from posterior compression by the muscles and fibrous tissue on the unprotected dura following to the craniectomy. The arachnoid preserving duraplasty was done with the intention to avoid CSF-related complications like CSF leak, pseudomeningocele and meningitis. Later, we thought of maintaining the newly formed CSF space by tenting the duraplasty with the cranioplasty. Initially, we used to put a titanium mesh as it is, but with time we faced some complications and started to shape the titanium mesh into the shape

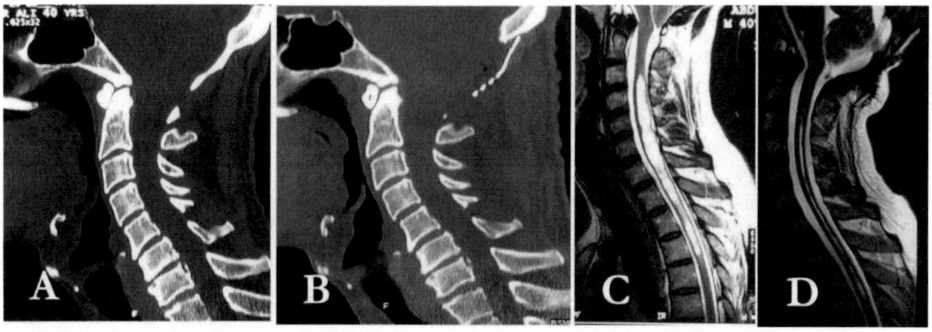

Figure 2.
Pre and postoperative images: (A) preoperative CT scan showing shallow posterior fossa and narrow foramen magnum, (B) postoperatively which has clearly increased in volume and diameter respectively, (C) preoperative MRI shows tonsillar herniation, absence of cisterna magna and big syrinx, and (D) postoperative MRI showing tonsillar ascent, appearance of good retrocerebellar CSF space and obvious resolution of syrinx.

of a Stealth bomber, thus we call it "Stealth cranioplasty". The Stealth cranioplasty can also prevent cerebellar slump as we flatten the upper portion to support the cerebellum. As a whole, we intended to increase the posterior fossa volume to restore and maintain normal anatomy and physiology around the foramen magnum including the CSF dynamics as well as to prevent cerebellar slump, CSF related complications and recurrence. Reduced financial and psychological burden on the patients came as a byproduct as they did not have complications and did not need any redo surgery so far. As of March 2019, we performed Stealth cranioplasty on 17 symptomatic adults for CM1 with SM and all are doing well without any complication or recurrence.

4. Final remarks and future directions

It was the Japanese neurosurgeons, who pioneered the cranioplasty for CM1. After that, quite a few attempts have been made to manage CM1 by cranioplasty in different formats. Even though, not a regular practice for CM1 surgery, cranioplasty can successfully be performed in selected cases with good outcome.

Different techniques of cranioplasty have been devised with different concepts. Whatever the strategy is preferred, the ultimate goal is to give CM1 patients the utmost benefit. Cranioplasty was first adopted with the aim to increase the volume of the posterior cranial fossa as most of the surgeons of this genre believe that the shallow posterior fossa is the main pathology behind development of CM1. The next other important pathology related to CM is the aberration of the CSF dynamics around the CVJ, which is also believed to be a consequence of the abnormal physiology resulting from the small posterior fossa. The cranioplasties also aim to manage this problem of CSF dynamics and with most of the cranioplasty procedures, this can be managed successfully. Apart from these two, the other valid objectives to choose cranioplasty in treatment of CM can be, dealing and preventing complications like cerebellar ptosis, dural ectasia, CSF related complications, post-surgery headaches and recurrences.

Till now, there is no common method for managing all cases of CM. Thus, every CM should be dealt with its individuality. The genetics of CM is being revealed now with time and the genetic basis of the pathophysiology of CM may allow scientists to manage all CM patients in a single manner in future. Until then, cranioplasty in different formats may serve as good means of dealing most of the straightforward cases of CM as the primary treatment modality in different combinations.

Cranioplasty can play effective role in addressing the primary pathology as well as the way to prevent and manage most of the possible complications. In general, this can be adopted as a routine procedure for most of the cases.

Acknowledgements

I am indebted to my colleagues and patients for their enormous support in so many ways in writing this chapter.

Conflict of interest

None.

Author details

Asifur Rahman
Department of Neurosurgery, Bangabandhu Sheikh Mujib Medical University, Dhaka, Bangladesh

*Address all correspondence to: bijoun14@yahoo.com

References

[1] Chiari H. Concerning alterations in the cerebellum resulting from cerebral hydrocephalus. Pediatric Neurosurgery. 1987;**13**(1):3-8

[2] Koehler P. Chiari's description of cerebellar ectopy (1891): With a summary of Cleland's and Arnold's contributions and some early observations on neural-tube defects. Journal of Neurosurgery. 1991;**75**(5):823-826

[3] Massimi L, Peppucci E, Peraio S, Di Rocco C. History of Chiari type I malformation. Neurological Sciences. 2011;**32**(3):263-265

[4] Pearce J. Arnold chiari, or "Cruveilhier cleland Chiari" malformation. Journal of Neurology, Neurosurgery & Psychiatry. 2000;**68**(1):13

[5] Carmel P, Markesbery W. Early descriptions of the Arnold-Chiari malformation. The contribution of John Cleland. Journal of Neurosurgery. 1972;**37**(5):543-547

[6] Fries FN, Hendrix P, Brinker TJ, Loukas M, Tubbs RS. Otto Mennicke (1876–) and the first description of skull base anomalies causing cerebellar tonsillar ectopia: One of the first mentions of the Chiari I malformation. Child's Nervous System. 2017;**33**(5):825-827

[7] Tubbs RS, Oakes WJ. The Chiari Malformations: A Historical Context. The Chiari Malformations. New York: Springer; 2013. pp. 5-11

[8] Alden TD, Ojemann JG, Park T. Surgical treatment of Chiari I malformation: Indications and approaches. Neurosurgical Focus. 2001;**11**(1):1-5

[9] Lee HS, Lee S-H, Kim ES, Kim J-S, Lee J-I, Shin HJ, et al. Surgical results of arachnoid-preserving posterior fossa decompression for Chiari I malformation with associated syringomyelia. Journal of Clinical Neuroscience. 2012;**19**(4):557-560

[10] Kennedy BC, Kelly KM, Phan MQ, Bruce SS, McDowell MM, Anderson RC, et al. Outcomes after suboccipital decompression without dural opening in children with Chiari malformation type I. Journal of Neurosurgery: Pediatrics. 2015;**16**(2):150-158

[11] Navarro R, Olavarria G, Seshadri R, Gonzales-Portillo G, McLone DG, Tomita T. Surgical results of posterior fossa decompression for patients with Chiari I malformation. Child's Nervous System. 2004;**20**(5):349-356

[12] Munshi I, Frim D, Stine-Reyes R, Weir BK, Hekmatpanah J, Brown F. Effects of posterior fossa decompression with and without duraplasty on Chiari malformation-associated hydromyelia. Neurosurgery. 2000;**46**(6):1384-1390

[13] Pomeraniec IJ, Ksendzovsky A, Awad AJ, Fezeu F, Jane JA. Natural and surgical history of Chiari malformation type I in the pediatric population. Journal of Neurosurgery: Pediatrics. 2016;**17**(3):343-352

[14] Quon JL, Grant RA, DiLuna ML. Multimodal evaluation of CSF dynamics following extradural decompression for Chiari malformation type I. Journal of Neurosurgery: Spine. 2015;**22**(6):622-630

[15] Gardner WJ, Goodall RJ. The surgical treatment of Arnold-Chiari malformation in adults: An explanation of its mechanism and importance of encephalography in diagnosis. Journal of Neurosurgery. 1950;7(3):199-206

[16] Krieger MD, McComb JG, Levy ML. Toward a simpler surgical

management of Chiari I malformation in a pediatric population. Pediatric Neurosurgery. 1999;**30**(3):113-121

[17] Kurzbuch AR, Jayamohan J, Magdum S. Decompressive surgery for Chiari I malformation in children without dural repair: A still effective and safe procedure? Child's Nervous System. 2019;**35**:1-8

[18] Badie B, Mendoza D, Batzdorf U. Posterior fossa volume and response to suboccipital decompression in patients with Chiari I malformation. Neurosurgery. 1995;**37**(2):214-218

[19] Batzdorf U, McArthur DL, Bentson JR. Surgical treatment of Chiari malformation with and without syringomyelia: Experience with 177 adult patients. Journal of Neurosurgery. 2013;**118**(2):232-242

[20] Bonney PA, Maurer AJ, Cheema AA, Duong Q, Glenn CA, Safavi-Abbasi S, et al. Clinical significance of changes in pB-C2 distance in patients with Chiari type I malformations following posterior fossa decompression: A single-institution experience. Journal of Neurosurgery: Pediatrics. 2016;**17**(3):336-342

[21] Cools MJ, Quinsey CS, Elton SW. Chiari decompression outcomes using ligamentum nuchae harvest and duraplasty in pediatric patients with Chiari malformation type I. Journal of Neurosurgery: Pediatrics. 2018;**22**(1):47-51

[22] Oral S, Yilmaz A, Kucuk A, Tumturk A, Menku A. Comparison of dural splitting and duraplasty in patients with Chiari type I malformation: Relationship between tonsillo-dural distance and syrinx cavity. Turkish Neurosurgery. 2019;**29**(2):229-236

[23] Radmanesh A, Greenberg JK, Chatterjee A, Smyth MD, Limbrick DD, Sharma A. Tonsillar pulsatility before and after surgical decompression for children with Chiari malformation type 1: An application for true fast imaging with steady state precession. Neuroradiology. 2015;**57**(4):387-393

[24] Singhal GD, Singhal S, Agrawal G, Singhal D, Arora V. Surgical experience in pediatric patients with Chiari-I malformations aged ≤ 18 years. Journal of Neurosciences in Rural Practice. 2019;**10**(1):85

[25] Hida K, Iwasaki Y, Koyanagi I, Sawamura Y, Abe H. Surgical indication and results of foramen magnum decompression versus syringosubarachnoid shunting for syringomyelia associated with Chiari I malformation. Neurosurgery. 1995;**37**(4):673-679

[26] Zhang L, Yi Z, Duan H, Li L. A novel autologous duraplasty in situ technique for the treatment of Chiari malformation type I. Journal of Neurosurgery. 2017;**126**(1):91-97

[27] Rahman A, Rana MS, Bhandari PB, Asif DS, Uddin ANW, Obaida ASMA, et al. "Stealth cranioplasty:" A novel endeavor for symptomatic adult Chiari I patients with syringomyelia: Technical note, appraisal, and philosophical considerations. Journal of Craniovertebral Junction and Spine. 2017;**8**(3):243

[28] Aghakhani N, Parker F, David P, Morar S, Lacroix C, Benoudiba F, et al. Long-term follow-up of Chiari-related syringomyelia in adults: Analysis of 157 surgically treated cases. Neurosurgery. 2009;**64**(2):308-315

[29] Alfieri A, Pinna G. Long-term results after posterior fossa decompression in syringomyelia with adult Chiari type I malformation. Journal of Neurosurgery: Spine. 2012;**17**(5):381-387

[30] Armonda RA, Citrin CM, Foley KT, Ellenbogen RG. Quantitative cine-mode

magnetic resonance imaging of Chiari I malformations: An analysis of cerebrospinal fluid dynamics. Neurosurgery. 1994;**35**(2):214-224

[31] Ladner TR, Dewan MC, Day MA, Shannon CN, Tomycz L, Tulipan N, et al. Evaluating the relationship of the pB-C2 line to clinical outcomes in a 15-year single-center cohort of pediatric Chiari I malformation. Journal of Neurosurgery: Pediatrics. 2015;**15**(2):178-188

[32] Batzdorf U. Chiari I malformation with syringomyelia: Evaluation of surgical therapy by magnetic resonance imaging. Journal of Neurosurgery. 1988;**68**(5):726-730

[33] Alzate JC, Kothbauer KF, Jallo GI, Epstein FJ. Treatment of Chiari type I malformation in patients with and without syringomyelia: A consecutive series of 66 cases. Neurosurgical Focus. 2001;**11**(1):1-9

[34] Stanko KM, Lee YM, Rios J, Wu A, Sobrinho GW, Weingart JD, et al. Improvement of syrinx resolution after tonsillar cautery in pediatric patients with Chiari type I malformation. Journal of Neurosurgery: Pediatrics. 2016;**17**(2):174-181

[35] Milhorat TH, Johnson WD, Miller JI, Bergland RM, Hollenberg-Sher J. Surgical treatment of syringomyelia based on magnetic resonance imaging criteria. Neurosurgery. 1992;**31**(2):231-245

[36] Rocque BG, Oakes WJ. Surgical treatment of Chiari I malformation. Neurosurgery Clinics. 2015;**26**(4):527-531

[37] Ratre S, Yadav N, Yadav YR, Parihar VS, Bajaj J, Kher Y. Endoscopic management of Arnold-Chiari malformation type I with or without syringomyelia. Journal of Neurological Surgery Part A: Central European Neurosurgery. 2018;**79**(01):045-051

[38] Zagzoog N, Reddy KK. Use of minimally invasive tubular retractors for foramen magnum decompression of Chiari malformation: A technical note and case series. World Neurosurgery. 2019;**128**:248-253

[39] Tokuno H, Suzuki T, Nishimura S, Hakuba A, editors. Operative treatment of Chiari malformation with syringomyelia. In: Proceedings of the 8th European Congress of Neurosurgery; September 6-11, 1987; Barcelona. Springer; 1988

[40] Sakamoto H, Nishikawa M, Hakuba A, Yasui T, Kitano S, Nakanishi N, et al. Expansive suboccipital cranioplasty for the treatment of syringomyelia associated with Chiari malformation. Acta Neurochirurgica. 1999;**141**(9):949-961

[41] Holly LT, Batzdorf U. Management of cerebellar ptosis following craniovertebral decompression for Chiari I malformation. Journal of Neurosurgery. 2001;**94**(1):21-26

[42] Di Rocco C, Velardi F. Acquired Chiari type I malformation managed by supratentorial cranial enlargement. Child's Nervous System. 2003;**19**(12):800-807

[43] Nishikawa M, Ohata K, Baba M, Terakawa Y, Hara M. Chiari I malformation associated with ventral compression and instability: One-stage posterior decompression and fusion with a new instrumentation technique. Neurosurgery. 2004;**54**(6):1430-1435

[44] Takayasu M, Nishizawa T, Yoshida J. Simple Expansive Suboccipital Cranioplasty Following Foramen Magnum Decompression for the Treatment of Syringomyelia Associated with Chiari I Malformation.

Syringomyelia: Springer; 2001. pp. 159-163

[45] Takayasu M, Takagi T, Hara M, Anzai M. A simple technique for expansive suboccipital cranioplasty following foramen magnum decompression for the treatment of syringomyelia associated with Chiari I malformation. Neurosurgical Review. 2004;**27**(3):173-177

[46] Itoh Y, Kuwahara N, Hirano Y, Sasajima T, Suzuki A, Mizoi K. Surgical Treatment of Syringomyelia Associated with Chiari I Malformation: Advantage of Cranioplasty Using Hydroxyapatite Implants. Syringomyelia: Springer; 2001. pp. 188-193

[47] Sheikh BY. Simple and safe method of cranial reconstruction after posterior fossa craniectomy. Surgical Neurology. 2006;**65**(1):63-66

[48] Heller JB, Lazareff J, Gabbay JS, Lam S, Kawamoto HK, Bradley JP. Posterior cranial fossa box expansion leads to resolution of symptomatic cerebellar ptosis following Chiari I malformation repair. The Journal of Craniofacial Surgery. 2007;**18**(2):274-280

[49] Di X, Luciano MG, Benzel EC. Acute respiratory arrest following partial suboccipital cranioplasty for cerebellar ptosis from Chiari malformation decompression: Report of 2 cases. Neurosurgical Focus. 2008;**25**(6):E12

[50] Chou Y-C, Sarkar R, Osuagwu FC, Lazareff JA. Suboccipital craniotomy in the surgical treatment of Chiari I malformation. Child's Nervous System. 2009;**25**(9):1111-1114

[51] Furtado SV, Anantharam BA, Reddy K, Hegde AS. Repair of Chiari III malformation using cranioplasty and an occipital rotation flap: Technical note and review of literature. Surgical Neurology. 2009;**72**(4):414-417

[52] Oró JJ, Mueller DM. Posterior fossa decompression and reconstruction in adolescents and adults with the Chiari I malformation. Neurological Research. 2011;**33**(3):261-271

[53] Bambakidis NC, Dickman CA. Surgery of the Craniovertebral Junction. New York: Thieme; 2012

[54] Assina R, Meleis AM, Cohen MA, Iqbal MO, Liu JK. Titanium mesh-assisted dural tenting for an expansile suboccipital cranioplasty in the treatment of Chiari 1 malformation. Journal of Clinical Neuroscience. 2014;**21**(9):1641-1646

[55] Choi J-I, Dhong ES, Lim D-J, Kim S-D. Reduction cranioplasty for macrocephaly with long-standing hydrocephalus and non-fused Fontanelle in Chiari malformation type I. Child's Nervous System. 2014;**30**(10):1763-1766

[56] Udani V, Holly LT, Chow D, Batzdorf U. Posterior fossa reconstruction using titanium plate for the treatment of cerebellar ptosis after decompression for Chiari malformation. World Neurosurgery. 2014;**81**(5-6):836-841

[57] Alsahlawi A, Ekhzaimy A, Alshowair D, Ajlan A. Decompressive cranioplasty in a patient with osteopetrosis. World Neurosurgery. 2017;**108**:991.e1-991.e5

[58] Korshunov A, Kushel Y. Expansive Suboccipital Cranioplasty in Chiari-1 Malformation (a Case Report and Technical Notes). Moscow: Media Sphera Publishing Group; 2017. p. 92

[59] Tjokorda GM, Tjokorda GS. A less invasive suboccipital decompression-cranioplasty for Chiari type I malformation: Is it beneficial? Interdisciplinary Neurosurgery. 2018;**14**:59-62

[60] Valentini LG, Saletti V, Erbetta A, Chiapparini L, Furlanetto M. Chiari 1 malformation and untreated sagittal synostosis: A new subset of complex Chiari? Child's Nervous System. 2019;**35**:1-13

Chapter 4

"Stealth Cranioplasty" for Adult Chiari Malformation Type 1: A Philosophical Journey of Innovation, Adaptation, and Evolution

Asifur Rahman

Abstract

Chiari malformation (CM) and its management are long debated enigmas for neurosurgeons. Many surgical procedures have been innovated and are in practice for this perplexing and daunting entity to give the patients a satisfactory remedy. But, a unanimously accepted surgical procedure is still lacking to achieve gratifying result. We tried to develop a novel technique, which we call the "stealth cranioplasty (SCP)," to help the adult Chiari malformation type 1 (CM1) patients. In this chapter, the philosophy behind developing the technique of "stealth cranioplasty" by reconstruction of posterior fossa (PF) by cranioplasty with pre-shaped titanium mesh is described. Different stages, difficulties, and modifications of the journey toward the present day status are also elaborated graphically.

Keywords: Chiari malformation, Chiari malformation type 1, arachnoid-preserving duraplasty, stealth cranioplasty, posterior fossa

1. Introduction

The baffling malady of Chiari malformation (CM) is still an enigma for neurosurgeons for its poorly understood pathophysiology, uncertain natural history, and dilemma concerning management options since Hans Chiari described it first in 1891 and detailed with refinements in 1896. Even being a diverse disease in presentation, Chiari malformation is being detected more often than before because of the advent of magnetic resonance imaging (MRI) and its better delineation of soft tissue especially in the posterior fossa (PF) and the craniovertebral junction (CVJ). Owing to its diverse presentations, varied thoughts on pathophysiology, and numerous philosophies in management, a myriad of surgical options are existent for CM. Better understanding of pathophysiology with technical advancements and better availability of imaging facilities have made CM more treatable with encouraging outcomes, and CM no more remains an unfamiliar entity. In this chapter we will present a novel technique that we developed over years to treat only the adult Chiari malformation type 1 (CM1) patients. We will also discuss about the philosophy behind developing this as well as the evolution process of the procedure focusing on the problems that we faced and how we modified our procedure to solve those and finally reached here. With our procedure we tried to address the two most common pathophysiological aspects of CM1 rationally that play the major roles: the shallow posterior fossa and the difference in pressure gradient of cerebrospinal fluid (CSF) between cranial and spinal compartments. With our procedure we also tried to prevent recurrence and avoid complications in a cost-effective way.

2. Pathophysiology

Any conclusive pathology in development of Chiari malformations is still lacking, and heterogeneity of theories regarding pathogenesis of CM continues to deepen the controversy. The most popular and accepted theory regarding Chiari 1 is that it is a developmental anomaly that causes tonsillar herniation from a discrepancy between the content, the hindbrain and the container, and the posterior fossa [1, 2]. Arguments can be made that this malady entirely is not a malformation. The shallow posterior fossa is an anomaly or deviation from the normal arrangement in its structure, while the herniation of the part of the normal hindbrain is an alteration that the nature makes in an attempt to maintain the homeostasis in the posterior fossa and the CVJ [3]. The origin of shallow PF may have several pathological bases, and our technique is primarily based on the theory of shallow posterior fossa as well as other pathologies that play important role in development of CM.

2.1 Evolution of human skull and brain and CM1

Studies on human evolution have revealed significant changes in the braincase; the skull, especially in the posterior skull base region; and the brain itself. Analysis on evolution demonstrated the gradual increase in cranial capacity from about 800 cm^3 in Homo erectus to 1000–1200 cm^3 in the species of the Middle Pleistocene and further to 1500 cm^3 in Neanderthals and modern humans [4–6]. But in the process of evolution from Homo neanderthalensis to *Homo sapiens*, both the cranial capacity and basal angle had decreased considerably, while the brain size increased significantly [5]. The posterior cranial fossa of *H. sapiens* has diminished in size, occupying around 26.8% of the available intracranial space, while in CM1 this space is further reduced to around 21.6%, resulting from different factors [7]. Modern human beings may carry some primitive genes of ancient hominins in their genomic code influenced by gene flow interchange, interbreeding, and anatomic reshaping of the skull base during evolution at random in some individuals of CM1 [5]. So, the shallow and small posterior fossa in CM1 may bear an evolutionary imprint.

2.2 Genetics of CM1

The majority of cases of CM1 are considered as sporadic. However, there are clues that suggest a genetic component playing role in development of Chiari in at least a subset of patients. Evidence of manifestation of CM1 in twins, in siblings, in first-degree relatives, in familial clustering among generations, or in conjunction with some known genetic syndromes supports the genetic origin vigorously. From these, it can be presumed that genetic factors, along with other epigenetic and/or environmental factors, prompt development of a small posterior cranial fossa. Familial aggregation is a representative of traits that hints to an underlying genetic basis [8–19]. Studies of families having Chiari among the members suggest posterior fossa volume (PFV) to be highly heritable, and genetic analysis reveals indicative linkage to regions at chromosomes 1q, 8q, 9q, 12p, 12q, 15q, and 22q. Moreover, disturbance in formation of the basichondrocranium from hyperossification or hypo-ossification has the possibility of having morphometric changes in the posterior cranial fossa in patients with Chiari resulting from the misregulation in genes [13, 20–24].

2.3 Embryological basis of CM1

In the development of a shallow and small posterior fossa, embryological derangement is pivotal. Occipitocervical transition develops during the fourth week of embryological life from bilateral four occipital somites (OS1–OS4) and seven cervical somites (CS1–CS7) that form the axial skeleton [25–27]. Different parts of the occipital bone originate from different somites and grow at different paces. This discrepancy in the rate of growth of different parts of the occipital bone during development leads to the typical developmental disorder of CM1 [28]. The supratentorial part of the squamous occipital derives from membranous origin, while the infratentorial part comes from cartilaginous origin. The shallowness of the posterior fossa may result from an abnormality of the lower part of the occipital squamous bone derived from the cartilaginous origin. The chondrified supraocciput, which is vulnerable to regression, theoretically offers an embryological basis for the shortening of the supraocciput in CM [29].

2.4 Posterior fossa volume and development of CM1

From the thoughtful observations and meticulous analysis, along with his theory of chronically raised intracranial pressure (ICP), Chiari furthermore believed that inadequate bone growth and insufficient enlargement of skull triggered raised ICP which plays a vital role in this condition to force down the hindbrain [30–33]. Cleland in 1883 and Mennicke in 1891 also advocated that the pathology lies in the defective bone around the foramen magnum while describing hindbrain herniation [34, 35]. Many studies in the modern era, with the help of modern technological advancements, have also strongly proven that the posterior fossa is indeed shallow or smaller than the normal hindbrain in Chiari patients. The shallowness of the posterior fossa has been proven in Chiari patients in comparison to controls using X-rays [36, 37]. Ratio of the posterior fossa with supratentorial volumes on MR images between patients with Chiari 1 malformation and controls also demonstrated smaller ratio in Chiari patients who were symptomatic, and most of them improved following posterior fossa decompression (PFD) [38].

Some studies found PFV to be smaller in pediatric CM1 patients also, which matches the studies in adults and aids the theory relating to the pathophysiological mechanism of CM1 resulting from small posterior fossa [7]. Interestingly, in cases of acquired Chiari malformation (ACM), surgical management of only the primary lesion has shown to improve ACM which also supports the discrepancy between the volume of the posterior fossa and its contents [39]. From different studies, it is now proposed that development of Chiari results from multifactorial etiologies, where small PF remains to be the most crucial one [40–52]. The theory of small PF is further strengthened by demonstration of CM by creating smaller basichondrocrania and posterior cranial fossa than controls by producing a state of hypervitaminosis A in experimental models of rodents [53]. Moreover, CM1 has been described in several metabolic disorders also like Paget's disease [54], rickets [55, 56], craniometaphyseal dysplasia [57], acromegaly [58], and growth hormone deficiency [59], where the PFV is rendered smaller than usual.

2.5 Tonsillar descent in CM1

By definition, radiologically, tonsillar herniation more than 5 mm below the foramen magnum is considered to be CM1. Incidental findings of patients having more than 5 mm descent of tonsil without any recognizable symptoms of Chiari are not uncommon. On the other hand, there are patients who have less than 5 mm descent of the tonsils and yet show pronounced symptoms of CM1. Though the cerebellar tonsillar herniation is the most commonly used radiological measurement to determine the diagnosis of CM1, clinical presentations often pose dilemma in decision making. So, this radiological measurement of degree of tonsillar descent alone may not be reliable enough to ascertain the presence and severity of CM1 and should always be tallied with the clinicopathological setting [1, 60–70].

2.6 Cranial and spinal cerebrospinal fluid pressure gradient difference in pathogenesis of CM1

Chiari, while describing the hindbrain herniation first, hypothesized the changes to be related to congenital hydrocephalus [30]. Studies later revealed that the malformation is not always accompanied by hydrocephalus; rather the fetal cerebellar herniation is due to the lowered intraspinal pressure owing to leakage of CSF at the myelocele, especially in cases of Chiari type 2 [71–74].

In fact, it is recommended that the pressure difference between the cranial and spinal compartments is the force responsible for the herniation. It is very much feasible as the brain tissue is a thick jelly like substance and acts like a viscoelastic medium to be subjected to deformation in response to stress [75]. Thus, any imbalance between the cranial and spinal CSF compartments leading to reduced CSF pressure in the spinal compartment may result in spontaneous occurrence of a CM1 which is also evidenced by tonsillar herniation following spinal shunting procedure. Conversion of a lumbar shunt to a ventricular shunt has shown to eliminate the downward craniospinal pressure gradient, leading to the reversal of the tonsillar descent or at least arresting further migration amplifying the aptness of this theory [74, 76–81]. This theory of disequilibrium of CSF dynamics might explain the reason of the tonsils to go back to their normal position following PFD which relieves the discrepancy of the pressure gradient between the cranial and spinal compartments, and our procedure is partly based on this theory also.

3. Commonly practiced surgical procedures

First attempted surgery for CM was in 1930 by a Dutchman Cornelis Joachimus Van Houweninge Graftdijk, on a patient with myelomeningocele and ventriculogram-proven hindbrain herniation. He tried surgically to relieve CSF obstruction at the CVJ by the redundant cerebellar tissue. His thought was to try to restore better flow of CSF by widening the space through which the brain had herniated [82]. For many years after the first attempt by Van Houweninge Graftdijk, surgery of CM carried grave prognosis. Now, with the better understanding of the pathology and improvements in technology, most patients with CM1 can be benefited by different surgical procedures [83].

Owing to the nature of this disorder and its diversity in clinical presentation and image findings, it is difficult to come to a consensus on which is the best way to manage this. Depending on presentation in milder forms of symptoms, some authors have advocated conservative management. However, according to most experts, surgical intervention remains the gold standard, both in reduction of tonsillar herniation, resolution of syrinx, and in overall outcome, in most of the cases [61, 66, 67, 84, 85]. The common procedure in almost all surgical approaches comprise of a suboccipital craniectomy with removal of posterior arch of C1 with the aim of posterior fossa decompression. Nevertheless, there are controversies concerning the extent of bone removal and additional measures taken along with it [86, 87]. Management of the dura includes leaving the dura intact with removal of the constricting band only [88], dural scoring [89, 90], resecting the outer layer of the dura [67, 91–94], opening the dura and leaving it open [95–98], and performing a duraplasty [38, 43, 67, 88, 91, 94, 99–104]. The arachnoid manipulation similarly varies from leaving it intact [88, 91, 105] to opening and resecting it [96, 99–103, 106, 107]. The cerebellar tonsils have been addressed in various ways also like not touching them [108], dissecting to separate them [99, 109], shrinking by bipolar coagulation [43, 67, 100, 102, 103, 110, 111], and subpial resection [38, 43, 67, 106, 107, 110, 112]. Recently, minimal invasive endoscopy-assisted decompression at the foramen magnum for CM has also been reported [113, 114].

4. Our technique

Many authors have postulated many factors to be responsible for development of Chiari malformations, and it seems that there actually are various pathologies in play. As the pathophysiology is multifactorial, it is almost impossible to address all the problems at a time with a single procedure. We tried to address the two basic pathologies that we feel to be of paramount importance in the pathophysiological process in the development of Chiari malformation. Accordingly we developed our technique only for the patients of CM1, which are young adults and do not have any other problem related to or complicating the condition like HCP, basilar invagination, and platybasia. Our patient subset also had syringes of different diameters and extensions. But we feel that it was not a big factor on influencing the result of the surgical technique, as the pathologies of both CM and SM seem to be the same. It was of our interest to see if the procedure addressing the Chiari only can solve syrinx as well, and that would provide some explanation that CM and SM share at least some common etiological factors and pathologies, which can be dealt with a single procedure.

Whatever theory regarding the pathophysiology is apt, with time and experience, centering on the two basic pathologies of shallow PF and imbalance of CSF dynamics around the CVJ, now the goal of our procedure is a persistent voluminous PF that would reestablish the CSF flow dynamics and would prevent recurrence and complications cost-effectively.

4.1 Patient positioning

We place the patient prone, in a modified concord position, under general anesthesia (**Figure 1A**). Special attention is given to keep the head in neutral position, and that is not flexed in any way. This gives two benefits. When the head is neutral, it helps the already jeopardized medulla from kinking from flexion as well as keeps it free from further compression by the herniated tonsils, which is already there. During reconstruction of the posterior fossa, neutral position gives better idea about the anatomy of the structures around the foramen magnum. This also gives the additional advantage of facilitation of venous return, by ensuring the jugular veins to be free of compression which helps in avoiding unnecessary oozing. Care of the airway, pressure points, and the vital monitoring are as usual.

4.2 Skin incision, harvesting graft, and exposure of bone

A midline skin incision is made from just above the external occipital protuberance down to a little below the prominence of the C2 vertebra. After opening the skin, a strip of the investing layer of the deep cervical fascia, measuring about 2 × 5 cm, is harvested for the duraplasty (**Figure 1B**). This strip is an advantageous graft material for duraplasty as it is autologous and hence can avoid foreign body reaction, potential risk of infection, and arachnoiditis. This graft is also flexible and durable. Most importantly, we do not need to make any additional wound to harvest it. Then the bones, up to the inion above and the posterior arch of the atlas below, are exposed by subperiosteal dissection maintaining the avascular plane in the midline along the ligamentum nuchae to reduce bleeding and postoperative pain from muscle injury. Subperiosteal dissection of the squamous occipital bone down to the margin of foramen magnum and the posterior arch of atlas is continued to expose the bones to a width of about 2 cm on each side.

4.3 Craniectomy

Two burr holes below the inion just lateral to the midline are made, and a 2.5–3 cm wide posterior fossa craniectomy is done in the midline extending from the foramen magnum to 4–5 cm above with the help of bone and Kerrison's rongeurs. Care is taken not to widen the craniectomy more than 1.5 cm beyond the midline on either side. In Chiari patients, often the bone around the inion is very thick. In those cases, the inner surface is undermined with the help of the Kerrison's rongeurs to make more space there. The posterior arch of the atlas is also removed about 1 cm on both sides of the midline (**Figure 1C**).

4.4 Dural opening and grafting

The dura is opened in the midline with a straight incision, keeping the arachnoid intact. On very rare occasions, there may be dural venous lakes or lacunae,

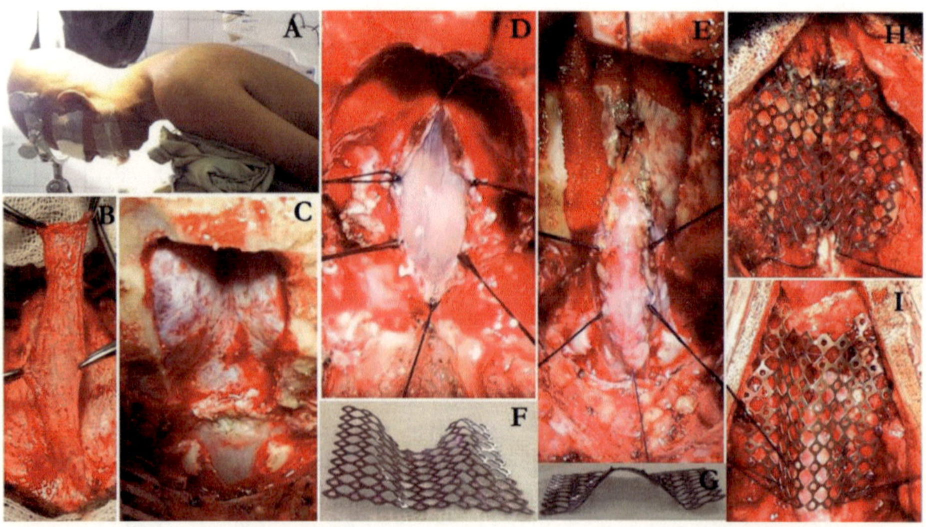

Figure 1.
Per-operative picture of different steps of stealth cranioplasty (SCP). Patient is placed prone with head in neutral position. (A) Harvesting of the cervical fascial graft. (B) Posterior fossa craniectomy is in the midline measuring 2.5–3.0 cm in width and 4–5 cm vertically from the foramen magnum. (C) Arachnoid-preserving midline dural opening and hitches for tenting. (D) Duraplasty with cervical fascial graft. (E) Molding of the titanium "stealth cranioplasty." (F and G) Fixing of the cranioplasty over the craniectomy gap. (H) Tenting of the duraplasty with the cranioplasty mesh (I).

which can be managed by continuous sutures along the cut margins to control the troublesome bleeding. If there is any accidental nick in the arachnoid, that is sealed with a very low bipolar cautery. The dural bands, which are present often, are kept as they are, to facilitate the dural tenting in the later part of the procedure. Two hitches are taken from the topmost and the lowermost points of the dural opening and two each from the free margins on either side. So, a total of six dural hitches are taken from the cut margins to tack those with the cranioplasty mesh later. The dural bands, which are not disturbed, help in strengthening the tenting where we want to pull the dura most, to widen the room in the posterior fossa around the foramen magnum (**Figure 1D**). The deep cervical fascial graft is sewn in the opening of the dura with 5–0 or 6–0 absorbable suture running stitches to complete an arachnoid-preserving duraplasty (APD) in a manner that when the dural tentings are fixed with the cranioplasty mesh, it resembles the roof of a hexagonal tent (**Figure 1E**).

4.5 Crafting of the stealth cranioplasty

The 5 × 5 cm titanium mesh (**Figure 2A**), which is malleable but tough enough to support the craniectomy gap after molding, is shaped to fit in the craniectomy gap in such a way that it covers the opening and at the same time increases the volume of the posterior fossa. The mesh is gradually curved in the middle like a longitudinally half-split cone, and the rest is kept flat (**Figures 1F, G** and **2B–F, H, I**). By this the half cone takes the contour of a cockpit, and the flat parts take the contour of the wings of a "stealth" bomber (**Figure 2G**). That's why we call it a "stealth cranioplasty". The tapered end of the half cone, which almost merges with the flat of the construct, is placed at the upper part of the craniectomy defect to fit with the curvature of the occipital bone near the occipital protuberance. The lower part of the molded mesh having the wider portion of the half cone is placed inferiorly. The margin of this broader edge of the cone is shaped in a manner of a half circle (**Figure 2E, F**), to create more space around the foramen magnum to provide more range of motion during neck extension postoperatively. The lower border of the wings of the cranioplasty is merged with the margin of the foramen magnum. The

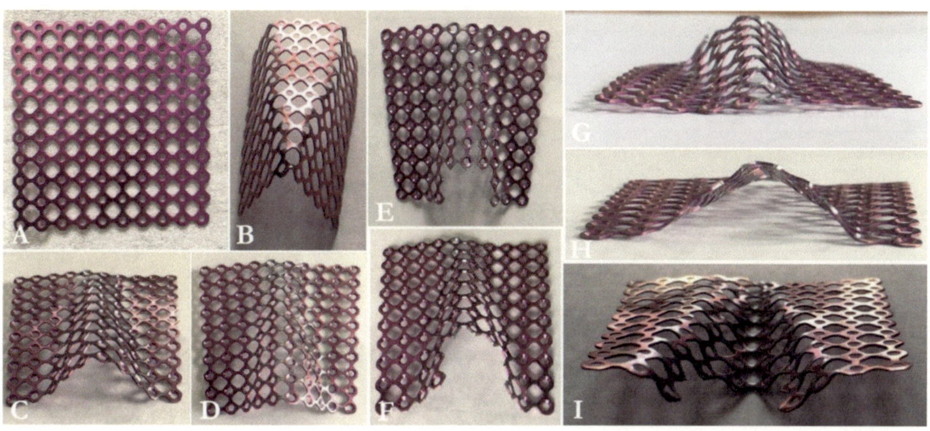

Figure 2.
Steps of molding of the titanium mesh to the shape of "stealth cranioplasty". The titanium mesh before molding. (A) The mesh is bent to make a triangular flat part in the middle. (B) The flat triangular part is curved into a longitudinally half split cone to mimic the cockpit and the sides are bent outwards to give them the contour of the wings of a Stealth bomber. (C & D) The widened part of the cone is cut in a crescent. (E & F) The pre-formed titanium mesh from front mimicking the cockpit of the Stealth bomber. (G) The look of the Stealth cranioplast from the wider part of the cone from rear (H) and below. (I).

rest of the wings is fixed with the bone at the lateral margins of the craniectomy defect to fit with the contour of the bone (**Figure 1H**).

4.6 Tenting and closure

The tentings are tied with the cranioplasty mesh to give the dural graft a final shape of the roof of a hexagonal tent (**Figure 1I**). Hemostasis is secured and the wound is closed in usual fashion in layers without any drain. Initially, there is some potential space between the dural graft and the cranioplasty, even after tenting. But this eventually is filled up with time by the pulsation of the brain as the duraplasty merges with the cranioplasty to create space for the CSF and neural structures.

5. Result

Eleven male and six female symptomatic CM1 adult patients, between age ranges of 22 and 42 years (mean 30.47 years), presented with different neurological symptoms related to CM1 and SM for 6–84 months (mean 27.70 months). The patients had syringes extending from three to more than ten vertebral levels (**Table 1**). All of the patients underwent PFD and arachnoid-preserving duraplasty followed by SCP and dural tenting and were followed up for a period of

Attribute	Number of patients (N = 17)
Gender	
Male	11
Female	6
Mean age in years (range)	30.47 (22–42 Years)
Clinical symptoms	
Sensory disturbance	12
Neck ache	10
Upper limb weakness	9
Lower limb weakness	6
Suboccipital headache	5
Duration of symptoms (months)	
1–12	3
13–24	4
25–36	3
37–48	4
49–60	2
>60	1
Extension of syrinx	
3–6 levels	6
7–10 levels	8
>10 levels	3

Table 1.
Showing distribution of gender, age, clinical symptoms, duration of symptoms, and extent of syrinx.

7–72 months (mean 32.59 months). Of 17 patients, 13 patients improved according to the Chicago Chiari Outcome Scale (CCOS) with score of 13–15, while 4 patients remained unchanged with CCOS of 12, and there was no worsening (**Table 2**). There was no complication related to Chiari surgery in any of the patients. All the patients had reestablishment of cisterna magna to different extents (**Figure 3E, F**). Five patients had marked reduction of syrinx, while 11 patients had moderate to mild reduction, and 1 patient had no change of syrinx. None of the patients needed redo surgery so far.

Parameters	Number of patients (N = 17)
Clinical outcome	
Improved	13
Unchanged	4
Worsened	0
CCOS	
13–16	13
9–12	4
<12	0
Radiological outcome of syrinx	
Marked reduction	5
Moderate reduction	7
Mild reduction	4
No reduction	1
Worsened/enlarged	0

Table 2.
Showing clinical outcome, outcome according to CCOS, and radiological outcome of syrinx.

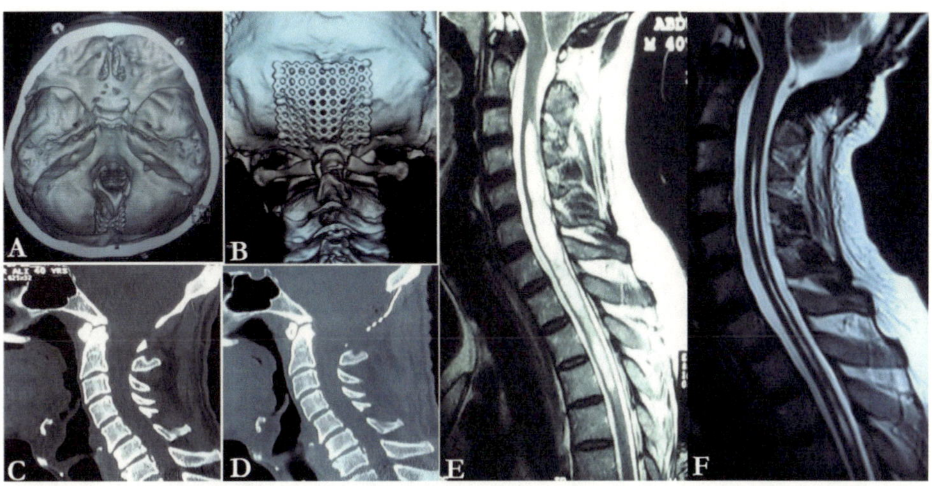

Figure 3.
Postoperative 3D CT scan following "stealth cranioplasty" increase in diameter of foramen magnum (A) and the final contour after fixing the cranioplasty with bone (B). Preoperative and (C) postoperative (D) sagittal reconstruction of bone around the CVJ showing increase in diameter of the foramen magnum and reconstruction of the posterior fossa in a shape of a sphere. Preoperative (E) and postoperative (F) sagittal T2WI ascent of the cerebellar tonsil, reestablishment of cisterna magna, and marked reduction of syrinx.

6. Our philosophy of innovation and evolution

Reconstruction of the posterior fossa by expansive cranioplasty is not practiced routinely following posterior fossa decompression for the CM1. Many authors have tried posterior fossa reconstruction with cranioplasty after PFD in many ways with different objectives. Cranioplasty as an attempt to treat and prevent further cerebellar subsidence during redo surgery has been described. Many techniques have been described in the literature like partial cranioplasty with methyl methacrylate (MMA) [115, 116], with autologous bone [117–122], and cranioplasty with different varieties of titanium prosthesis [48, 123–126]. Tacking of duraplasty with or without cranioplasty has also been described by some authors with intention to keep the cistern patent and to prevent adhesion [48, 120, 122, 123, 127]. We have tried to blend the procedures in an effective and least invasive way to give the utmost benefit to the patients.

Our journey began with the thought of the big concern of recurrence of symptoms in management of CM1. Postoperative recurrence of compression over the cerebellar tonsils around the foramen magnum and obliteration of CSF flow and dynamics around the CVJ may be caused by compression over the dura through the craniectomy gap by repositioned muscle bulk, fibrosis, and cerebellar sag.

We felt that, in conventional procedures, there is no measure to protect the dura from compression by the muscle bulk postoperatively from the back (**Figure 4A–C**). Initially the goal of cranioplasty was to prevent this by covering the craniectomy gap. Eventually, we felt that this cranioplasty can serve as a means to increase the posterior fossa volume as well.

So, we developed the technique based on our observations and thoughts in addition to the initial considerations of merely preventing recurrence and augmenting the posterior fossa volume.

Firstly, many patients come back with recurrences of symptoms from compression of the neuronal elements as well as obliteration of posterior CSF column by muscle bulk and fibrous tissue from posterior aspect around the surgical site as evident in many follow-up MRIs. This seemed to be due to having no protection against

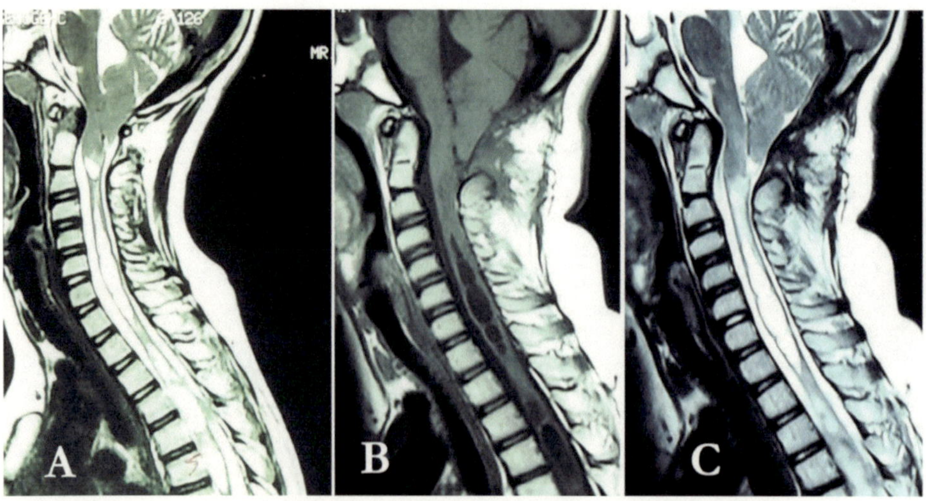

Figure 4.
Preoperative sagittal T2WI of a patient with CM1 and syrinx (A) 1 year postoperative sagittal T1WI and T2WI following posterior fossa bony decompression only. Worthy to note the posterior compression on dura by muscle and fibrous tissue and the status of Chiari and syrinx (B and C).

recompression from the posterior aspect. This led us to think about cranioplasty to make a protective safeguard against any compression from posterior aspect to avoid recurrence of symptoms.

Secondly, we wanted to augment the PFV so that the herniated contents can come back, can be accommodated with ease in the newly formed abode, and can relieve the compression around the foramen magnum to get the anatomy and physiology including CSF dynamics back to near normal. Any container which is spherical is more voluminous compared to a flat one. The pathology in case of CM1, is the shallow posterior fossa due to flattening of the lower part. Our endeavor is to make the posterior fossa more spherical and voluminous by performing the APD, SCP, and dural tenting.

Thirdly, cerebellar slump is often encountered when a larger craniectomy is done. This might be due to release of pressure in the posterior fossa creating much space, and the slump can further be aided by gravity. Though we do not make the craniectomy bigger than 2.5 cm wide and 3–4 cm vertically, this cranioplasty helps in preventing the cerebellar ptosis, even if there is any chance at all.

Fourthly, arachnoid-preserving duraplasty has the advantage of preventing postoperative arachnoiditis related to surgery which may result from manipulation of the arachnoid and seepage of blood into the subarachnoid space. APD also has the advantage of avoiding CSF-related complications. As the Pascal's law states, any force in a closed fluid filled container is equally distributed to all directions with the same force. Our hypothesis is that the force of CSF in the new space, aided by brain pulsation, is capable of opening up any adhesion of the arachnoid or creating new pathway naturally if ample space can be created. Some reports are there that sometimes there are arachnoid veils over the foramen of Magendie to block the CSF flow, and we are afraid that in this subset of patients, the SCP might not work to reestablish the CSF flow. Possibly there was no patient like this in our series, as we found all our patients to have better CSF flow around the CVJ. Moreover, as the bigger CSF space is molded and maintained around the CVJ by APD and dural tenting, the CSF makes its way to the spinal subarachnoid space to equilibrate the pressure gradient with the cranial CSF. This CSF equilibrium has the potential to push the tonsils up, back to the newly formed space, and keeps it floating with the buoyancy to prevent it from going down again and castoffs the need to handle the tonsils as well. Initially the new space is enlarged moderately to relieve the symptoms. With time and CSF pulsation, the space expands more and takes the contour of the cranioplasty and is maintained very well, making the PFV and CSF dynamics adequate to sustain relief of symptoms. Following PFD, APD, dural tenting, and SCP, with reversal of CSF dynamics to normalcy, the syrinx usually reduces without taking any additional measure. However, in a good number of cases, the syrinx takes a long time to resolve or does not resolve appreciably, and the symptoms related to syrinx resolve markedly.

Fifthly, with the APD with autologous fascia and hexagonal tacking of that with the "stealth" cranioplasty, some complications can be prevented effectively. The CSF-related complications like CSF leak, meningitis or pseudomeningocele, inflammation, scarring and adhesion of dural graft, cerebellar sag, and compression from behind can be avoided and prevented efficiently with this combined technique. The dural tacking can help in enhancing and maintaining the CSF space also.

Finally, financial and psychological burden other than physical disability takes a heavy toll on the patients of CM1 and their families. These financial and psychological burdens can be avoided as this is well affordable by the patients of a low socioeconomic condition like ours since it costs no more than USD $50 for the implant. At the same time, with this minimal expense, patients can avoid further extra expenses from re-surgery and rehabilitation program.

But all these adaptations did not take place straightway. We had to develop it step by step after facing different problems at different stages. Initially we had the considerations in mind that we have mentioned already. We started cranioplasty first with autologous bone with a titanium mesh buttress across the bone margins (**Figure 5A, B**). After few cases, we wanted to make it convenient for us by doing the cranioplasty with bone cement (MMA) with a buttress like the one as in cranioplasty with autologous bone (**Figure 5C, D**). We thought that the procedure can be made easier if we do the cranioplasty straight forward with a titanium mesh (**Figure 5E, F**). We expected that the gap created between the dura and the mesh by removing the bone at the craniectomy would be specious enough to serve the purpose of creating space for the cerebellum and reestablishment of CSF flow. That far we used to remove the dural bands only and did the cranioplasty with mesh and did so with satisfactory results in the next few cases until we faced problem with one patient 3 months postoperatively. This male patient was doing well postoperatively with marked improvement till he sneezed one morning and suddenly became quadriparetic. MRI showed greater herniation of the tonsils again (**Figure 6A, C**), while the immediate postop CT after the first surgery showed some ascent of the tonsil (**Figure 6A, B**). Preoperatively at the second surgery, we found that the dura was severely compressed along the lower margin of the mesh, and it seemed that the mesh margin has trapped the tonsil which was also evident in the MRI (**Figure 6C, D**). We only cut the inferior margin of the mesh in a crescentic shape and resected some fibrous tissue over the dura longitudinally to relieve the tonsils (**Figure 6E, F**), and the patient improved gradually. However the improvement was slow and was never as good as the first postoperative status.

After this, we routinely put the mesh by cutting the lower margin to make more space around the foramen magnum (**Figure 7A, B**). Then we thought that we can make some more space in the midline if we bend the mesh in the middle like a longitudinally half-split tube in the middle (**Figure 7C, D**). At this part of the advance of our journey, we started arachnoid-preserving duraplasty and dural tenting as well, and

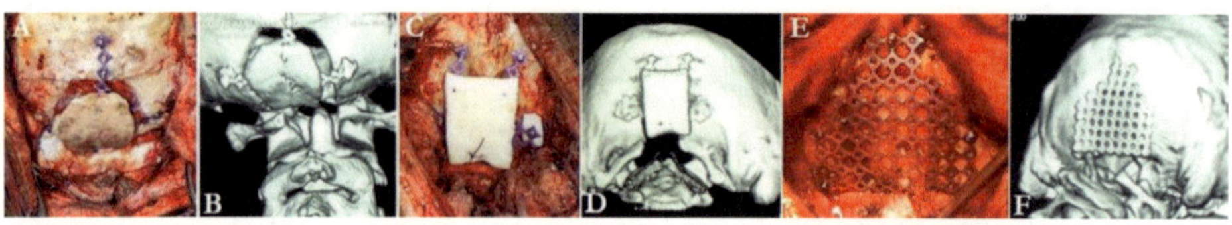

Figure 5.
Preoperative picture and postoperative 3D CT scan of cranioplasties using different materials. Cranioplasty with autologous bone (A and B), bone cement (MMA) (C and D), and flat titanium mesh (E and F).

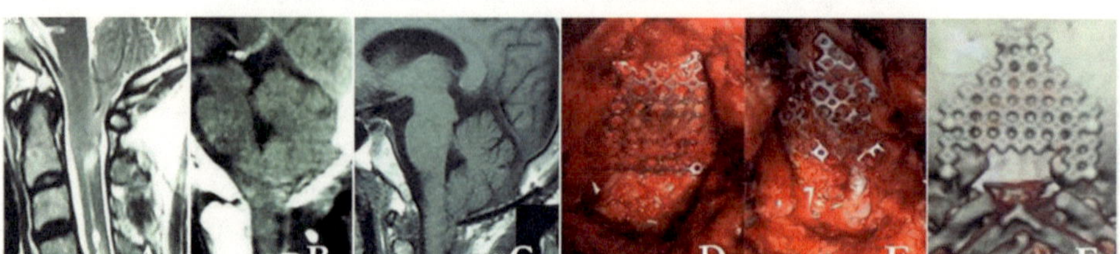

Figure 6.
MRI before first surgery of the patient that gave us the impetus to develop this technique, showing tonsillar herniation (A), CT scan after first surgery showing appreciable ascent of the tonsil (B), MRI before second surgery (after clinical deterioration) showing entrapped tonsil by the lower margin of the titanium mesh (C), preoperative picture at second surgery showing the dural compression by the lower margin of the titanium mesh (D), decompressed dura following cutting the lower margin of the titanium mesh and lysis of fibrosis (E), post of 3D CT scan to showing the lower cut margin of the titanium mesh to relieve the compression around the CVJ.

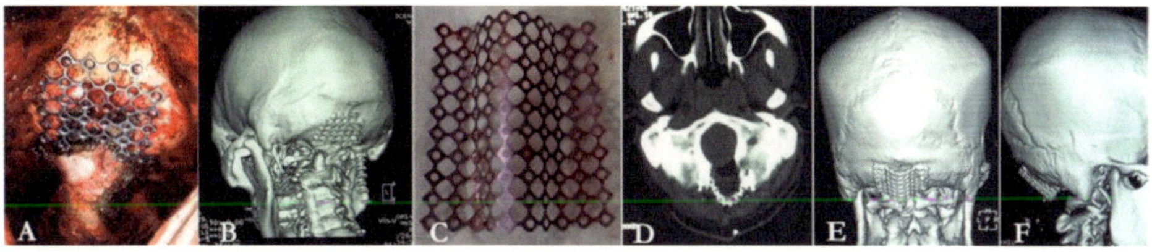

Figure 7.
Preoperative picture (A) and postoperative 3D CT scan (B) showing the placement of flat titanium mesh by cutting the lower margin to make more space around the foramen magnum. Molding of the titanium mesh in a longitudinally split half tube (C) which gives ample space around the foramen magnum as seen in postoperative CT scan (D). Postoperative 3D CT scan showing the protrusion around the external occipital protuberance (E and F).

that produced good results. We had to rethink of the shape of the mesh while molding, when some patients complained of some uneasiness from the little swelling under the skin from the bend at the upper part. Though we tried to merge the upper part of the tube-like bending with the external occipital protuberance, in some patients it was little more protruded than the external occipital protuberance (**Figure 7E, F**). We were afraid of skin excoriation in these patients after we were noticed about this problem. However, practically it did not produce any complication in any of the patients. We then changed the molding a little to come to the present day shape to merge the upper part with the bone near the external occipital protuberance by bending it like a longitudinally half split cone instead of a half split tube, which when fixed with the bone becomes flattened to merge with the contour of the occipital bone. Actually that gave us an additional benefit of preventing cerebellar sag also; as the upper part is flatter, this has more chance of supporting the cerebellum from sagging, if there is any chance at all through the narrow craniectomy gap (**Figure 3B**). This also gives the scope to increase the diameter of the foramen magnum (**Figure 3A, C, D**).

Treatment for CM1 is surgical and success of surgery depends on appropriate patient selection. We consider it a factor of paramount importance while selecting patients for stealth cranioplasty. Our patients are all adults, having no associated complex pathologies like hydrocephalus, platybasia, or basilar invagination, which gives us satisfactory result.

7. Conclusion

The journey to develop "stealth cranioplasty" was not a smooth one. After a lot of trial and error, now it seems to be an effective, fruitful, and cost-effective technique for management of symptomatic adult Chiari malformation type 1 with syringomyelia. This technique has the advantages of preventing complications and recurrences in addition to improvement of symptoms by addressing the basic pathology.

Acknowledgements

I am deeply indebted to the members of the team and sincerely thank them all for helping me in developing this technique with their valuable technical advices.

Conflict of interest

None.

Abbreviations

ACM	Acquired Chiari Malformation
APD	Arachnoid-preserving duraplasty
CCOS	Chicago Chiari Outcome Scale
CM	Chiari malformation
CM1	Chiari malformation type 1
CSF	Cerebrospinal fluid
CVJ	Craniovertebral junction
ICP	Intracranial pressure
MMA	Methyl methacrylate
MRI	Magnetic resonance imaging
PF	Posterior fossa
PFD	Posterior fossa decompression
PFV	Posterior fossa volume
SCP	Stealth cranioplasty
SM	Syringomyelia

Author details

Asifur Rahman
Department of Neurosurgery, Bangabandhu Sheikh Mujib Medical University, Shahbag, Dhaka, Bangladesh

*Address all correspondence to: bijoun14@yahoo.com

References

[1] Bejjani GK. Definition of the adult Chiari malformation: A brief historical overview. Neurosurgical Focus. 2001;**11**(1):1-8

[2] Poretti A, Ashmawy R, Garzon-Muvdi T, Jallo GI, Huisman TA, Raybaud C. Chiari type 1 deformity in children: Pathogenetic, clinical, neuroimaging, and management aspects. Neuropediatrics. 2016;**47**(05):293-307

[3] Rahman A. "Formation" of Chiari "malformation:" Nature's philosophical way of adaptation. Journal of Craniovertebral Junction and Spine. 2017;**8**(3):291

[4] Bruner E. Cranial shape and size variation in human evolution: Structural and functional perspectives. Child's Nervous System. 2007;**23**(12):1357-1365

[5] Fernandes YB, Ramina R, Campos-Herrera CR, Borges G. Evolutionary hypothesis for Chiari type I malformation. Medical Hypotheses. 2013;**81**(4):715-719

[6] Rightmire GP. Brain size and encephalization in early to mid-Pleistocene homo. American Journal of Physical Anthropology. 2004;**124**(2):109-123

[7] Furtado SV, Reddy K, Hegde A. Posterior fossa morphometry in symptomatic pediatric and adult Chiari I malformation. Journal of Clinical Neuroscience. 2009;**16**(11):1449-1454

[8] Atkinson JL, Kokmen E, Miller GM. Evidence of posterior fossa hypoplasia in the familial variant of adult Chiari I malformation: Case report. Neurosurgery. 1998;**42**(2):401-404

[9] Markunas CA, Tubbs RS, Moftakhar R, Ashley-Koch AE, Gregory SG, Oakes WJ, et al. Clinical, radiological, and genetic similarities between patients with Chiari type I and type 0 malformations. Journal of Neurosurgery: Pediatrics. 2012;**9**(4):372-378

[10] Mavinkurve GG, Sciubba D, Amundson E, Jallo GI. Familial Chiari type I malformation with syringomyelia in two siblings: Case report and review of the literature. Child's Nervous System. 2005;**21**(11):955-959

[11] Milhorat TH, Chou MW, Trinidad EM, Kula RW, Mandell M, Wolpert C, et al. Chiari I malformation redefined: Clinical and radiographic findings for 364 symptomatic patients. Neurosurgery. 1999;**44**(5):1005-1017

[12] Nagy L, Mobley J, Ray C. Familial aggregation of chiari malformation: Presentation, pedigree, and review of the literature. Turkish Neurosurgery. 2016;**26**(2):315-320

[13] Schanker BD, Walcott BP, Nahed BV, Kahle KT, Li YM, Coumans J-VC. Familial Chiari malformation: Case series. Neurosurgical Focus. 2011;**31**(3):E1

[14] Speer MC, George TM, Enterline DS, Franklin A, Wolpert CM, Milhorat TH. A genetic hypothesis for Chiari I malformation with or without syringomyelia. Neurosurgical Focus. 2000;**8**(3):1-4

[15] Stovner LJ, Cappelen J, Nilsen G, Sjaastad O. The Chiari type I malformation in two monozygotic twins and first-degree relatives. Annals of Neurology. 1992;**31**(2):220-222

[16] Szewka AJ, Walsh LE, Boaz JC, Carvalho KS, Golomb MR. Chiari in the family: Inheritance of the Chiari I malformation. Pediatric Neurology. 2006;**34**(6):481-485

[17] Tubbs RS, Hill M, Loukas M, Shoja MM, Oakes WJ. Volumetric analysis of the posterior cranial fossa in a family with four generations of the Chiari malformation type I. Journal of Neurosurgery: Pediatrics. 2008;**1**(1):21-24

[18] Turgut M. Chiari type I malformation in two monozygotic twins. British Journal of Neurosurgery. 2001;**15**(3):279-280

[19] Weisfeld-Adams JD, Carter MR, Likeman MJ, Rankin J. Three sisters with Chiari I malformation with and without associated syringomyelia. Pediatric Neurosurgery. 2007;**43**(6):533-538

[20] Boyles AL, Enterline DS, Hammock PH, Siegel DG, Slifer SH, Mehltretter L, et al. Phenotypic definition of Chiari type I malformation coupled with high-density SNP genome screen shows significant evidence for linkage to regions on chromosomes 9 and 15. American Journal of Medical Genetics Part A. 2006;**140**(24):2776-2785

[21] Markunas CA, Enterline DS, Dunlap K, Soldano K, Cope H, Stajich J, et al. Genetic evaluation and application of posterior cranial fossa traits as endophenotypes for Chiari type I malformation. Annals of Human Genetics. 2014;**78**(1):1-12

[22] Musolf AM, Ho WS, Long KA, Zhuang Z, Argersinger DP, Sun H, et al. Small posterior fossa in Chiari I malformation affected families is significantly linked to 1q43-44 and 12q23-24.11 using whole exome sequencing. European Journal of Human Genetics. 2019;**27**(10):1599-1610

[23] Sekula RF, Arnone GD, Crocker C, Aziz KM, Alperin N. The pathogenesis of Chiari I malformation and syringomyelia. Neurological Research. 2011;**33**(3):232-239

[24] Speer MC, Enterline DS, Mehltretter L, Hammock P, Joseph J, Dickerson M, et al. Chiari type I malformation with or without syringomyelia: Prevalence and genetics. Journal of Genetic Counseling. 2003;**12**(4):297-311

[25] Cambronero F, Puelles L. Rostrocaudal nuclear relationships in the avian medulla oblongata: A fate map with quail chick chimeras. The Journal of Comparative Neurology. 2000;**427**(4):522-545

[26] Carstens MH. Neural tube programming and the pathogenesis of craniofacial clefts, part I: The neuromeric organization of the head and neck. Handbook of Clinical Neurology. 2007;**87**:247-276

[27] Pang D, Thompson DN. Embryology and bony malformations of the craniovertebral junction. Child's Nervous System. 2011;**27**(4): 523-564

[28] Raybaud C, Jallo GI. Chiari 1 deformity in children: Etiopathogenesis and radiologic diagnosis. Handbook of Clinical Neurology. 2018;**155**:25-48. Elsevier

[29] Shoja MM, Ramdhan R, Jensen CJ, Chern JJ, Oakes WJ, Tubbs RS. Embryology of the craniocervical junction and posterior cranial fossa, part I: Development of the upper vertebrae and skull. Clinical Anatomy. 2018;**31**(4):466-487

[30] Chiari H. Concerning alterations in the cerebellum resulting from cerebral hydrocephalus. Pediatric Neurosurgery. 1987;**13**(1):3-8

[31] Koehler P. Chiari's description of cerebellar ectopy (1891): With a summary of Cleland's and Arnold's contributions and some early observations on neural-tube

defects. Journal of Neurosurgery. 1991;**75**(5):823-826

[32] Massimi L, Peppucci E, Peraio S, Di Rocco C. History of Chiari type I malformation. Neurological Sciences. 2011;**32**(3):263-265

[33] Pearce J. Arnold Chiari, or "Cruveilhier cleland Chiari" malformation. Journal of Neurology, Neurosurgery & Psychiatry. 2000;**68**(1):13

[34] Carmel P, Markesbery W. Early descriptions of the Arnold-Chiari malformation. The contribution of John Cleland. Journal of Neurosurgery. 1972;**37**(5):543-547

[35] Fries FN, Hendrix P, Brinker TJ, Loukas M, Tubbs RS. Otto Mennicke (1876–) and the first description of skull base anomalies causing cerebellar tonsillar ectopia: One of the first mentions of the Chiari I malformation. Child's Nervous System. 2017;**33**(5):825-827

[36] Nyland H, Krogness K. Size of posterior fossa in Chiari type 1 malformation in adults. Acta Neurochirurgica. 1978;**40**(3-4): 233-242

[37] Stovner L, Bergan U, Nilsen G, Sjaastad O. Posterior cranial fossa dimensions in the Chiari I malformation: Relation to pathogenesis and clinical presentation. Neuroradiology. 1993;**35**(2):113-118

[38] Badie B, Mendoza D, Batzdorf U. Posterior fossa volume and response to suboccipital decompression in patients with Chiari I malformation. Neurosurgery. 1995;**37**(2):214-218

[39] Wang J, Alotaibi NM, Samuel N, Ibrahim GM, Fallah A, Cusimano MD. Acquired Chiari malformation and syringomyelia secondary to space-occupying lesions: A systematic review. World Neurosurgery. 2017;**98**:800-808.e2

[40] Alkoç OA, Songur A, Eser O, Toktas M, Gönül Y, Esi E, et al. Stereological and morphometric analysis of MRI Chiari malformation type-1. Journal of Korean Neurosurgical Society. 2015;**58**(5):454

[41] Alperin N, Loftus JR, Oliu CJ, Bagci AM, Lee SH, Ertl-Wagner B, et al. Magnetic resonance imaging measures of posterior cranial fossa morphology and cerebrospinal fluid physiology in Chiari malformation type I. Neurosurgery. 2014;**75**(5):515-522

[42] Aydin S, Hanimoglu H, Tanriverdi T, Yentur E, Kaynar MY. Chiari type I malformations in adults: A morphometric analysis of the posterior cranial fossa. Surgical Neurology. 2005;**64**(3):237-241

[43] Batzdorf U, McArthur DL, Bentson JR. Surgical treatment of Chiari malformation with and without syringomyelia: Experience with 177 adult patients. Journal of Neurosurgery. 2013;**118**(2):232-242

[44] Biswas D, Eppelheimer MS, Houston JR, Ibrahimy A, Bapuraj JR, Labuda R, et al. Quantification of cerebellar crowding in type I Chiari malformation. Annals of Biomedical Engineering. 2019;**47**(3):731-743

[45] Dagtekin A, Avci E, Kara E, Uzmansel D, Dagtekin O, Koseoglu A, et al. Posterior cranial fossa morphometry in symptomatic adult Chiari I malformation patients: Comparative clinical and anatomical study. Clinical Neurology and Neurosurgery. 2011;**113**(5):399-403

[46] Greitz D, Wirestam R, Franck A, Nordell B, Thomsen C, Ståhlberg F. Pulsatile brain movement and associated

hydrodynamics studied by magnetic resonance phase imaging. Neuroradiology. 1992;**34**(5):370-380

[47] Karagöz F, Izgi N, Sencer SK. Morphometric measurements of the cranium in patients with Chiari type I malformation and comparison with the normal population. Acta Neurochirurgica. 2002;**144**(2):165-171

[48] Leung V, Magnussen JS, Stoodley MA, Bilston LE. Cerebellar and hindbrain motion in Chiari malformation with and without syringomyelia. Journal of Neurosurgery: Spine. 2016;**24**(4):546-555

[49] Noudel R, Jovenin N, Eap C, Scherpereel B, Pierot L, Rousseaux P. Incidence of basioccipital hypoplasia in Chiari malformation type I: Comparative morphometric study of the posterior cranial fossa. Journal of Neurosurgery. 2009;**111**(5):1046-1052

[50] Sgouros S, Kountouri M, Natarajan K. Posterior fossa volume in children with Chiari malformation type I. Journal of Neurosurgery: Pediatrics. 2006;**105**(2):101-106

[51] Shoja MM, Johal J, Oakes WJ, Tubbs RS. Embryology and pathophysiology of the Chiari I and II malformations: A comprehensive review. Clinical Anatomy. 2018;**31**(2):202-215

[52] Vega A, Quintana F, Berciano J. Basichondrocranium anomalies in adult Chiari type I malformation: A morphometric study. Journal of the Neurological Sciences. 1990;**99**(2-3):137-145

[53] Marin-Padilla M, Marin-Padilla TM. Morphogenesis of experimentally induced Arnold-Chiari malformation. Journal of the Neurological Sciences. 1981;**50**(1):29-55

[54] Richards PS, Bargiota A, Corrall RJ. Paget's disease causing an Arnold-Chiari type 1 malformation: Radiographic findings. American Journal of Roentgenology. 2001;**176**(3):816-817

[55] Caldemeyer KS, Boaz JC, Wappner RS, Moran CC, Smith RR, Quets JP. Chiari I malformation: Association with hypophosphatemic rickets and MR imaging appearance. Radiology. 1995;**195**(3):733-738

[56] Kuether TA, Piatt JH. Chiari malformation associated with vitamin D-resistant rickets: Case report. Neurosurgery. 1998;**42**(5):1168-1171

[57] Day RA, Park TS, Ojemann JG, Kaufman BA. Foramen magnum decompression for cervicomedullary encroachment in craniometaphyseal dysplasia: Case report. Neurosurgery. 1997;**41**(4):960-964

[58] Lemar JH, Perloff J, Merenich J. Symptomatic Chiari-I malformation in a patient with acromegaly. Southern Medical Journal. 1994;**87**(2):284-285

[59] Tubbs RS, Wellons JC III, Smyth MD, Bartolucci AA, Blount JP, Oakes WJ, et al. Children with growth hormone deficiency and Chiari I malformation: A morphometric analysis of the posterior cranial fossa. Pediatric Neurosurgery. 2003;**38**(6):324-328

[60] Aboulezz AO, Sartor K, Geyer CA, Gado MH. Position of cerebellar tonsils in the normal population and in patients with Chiari malformation: A quantitative approach with MR imaging. Journal of Computer Assisted Tomography. 1985;**9**(6):1033-1036

[61] Benglis D, Covington D, Bhatia R, Bhatia S, Elhammady MS, Ragheb J, et al. Outcomes in pediatric patients with Chiari malformation type I followed up without surgery. Journal of Neurosurgery: Pediatrics. 2011;7(4):375-379

[62] Elster AD, Chen M. Chiari I malformations: clinical and

radiologic reappraisal. Radiology. 1992;**183**(2):347-353

[63] Işik N, Elmaci I, Silav G, Celik M, Kalelioğlu M. Chiari malformation type III and results of surgery: A clinical study. Pediatric Neurosurgery. 2009;**45**(1):19-28

[64] Khalsa SSS, Geh N, Martin BA, Allen PA, Strahle J, Loth F, et al. Morphometricandvolumetriccomparison of 102 children with symptomatic and asymptomatic Chiari malformation type I. Journal of Neurosurgery: Pediatrics. 2018;**21**(1):65-71

[65] Meadows J, Kraut M, Guarnieri M, Haroun RI, Carson BS. Asymptomatic Chiari type I malformations identified on magnetic resonance imaging. Journal of Neurosurgery. 2000;**92**(6):920-926

[66] Novegno F, Caldarelli M, Massa A, Chieffo D, Massimi L, Pettorini B, et al. The natural history of the Chiari type I anomaly. Journal of Neurosurgery: Pediatrics. 2008;**2**(3):179-187

[67] Pomeraniec IJ, Ksendzovsky A, Awad AJ, Fezeu F, Jane JA. Natural and surgical history of Chiari malformation type I in the pediatric population. Journal of Neurosurgery: Pediatrics. 2016;**17**(3):343-352

[68] Sekula RF, Jannetta PJ, Casey KF, Marchan EM, Sekula LK, McCrady CS. Dimensions of the posterior fossa in patients symptomatic for Chiari I malformation but without cerebellar tonsillar descent. Cerebrospinal Fluid Research. 2005;**2**(1):11

[69] Shehu B, Ismail N, Mahmu M, Hassan I. Chiari I malformation: A missed diagnosis. Annals of African Medicine. 2006;**5**(4):206-208

[70] Smith BW, Strahle J, Bapuraj JR, Muraszko KM, Garton HJ, Maher CO. Distribution of cerebellar tonsil position: Implications for understanding Chiari malformation. Journal of Neurosurgery. 2013;**119**(3):812-819

[71] Cameron A. The Arnold-Chiari and other neuro-anatomical malformations associated with spina bifida. The Journal of Pathology and Bacteriology. 1957;**73**(1):195-211

[72] Emery JL, MacKenzie N. Medullo-cervical dislocation deformity (Chiari II deformity) related to neurospinal dysraphism (meningomyelocele). Brain. 1973;**96**(1):155-162

[73] van Hoy tenia G, Van den Berg R. Embryological studies of the posterior fossa in connection with Arnold-Chiari malformation. Developmental Medicine and Child Neurology. 1966;**8**:61-76

[74] Welch K, Shillito J, Strand R, Fischer EG, Winston KR. Chiari I "malformation"—An acquired disorder? Journal of Neurosurgery. 1981;**55**(4):604-609

[75] Fischer EG, Welch K, Shillito J. Syringomyelia following lumboureteral shunting for communicating hydrocephalus: Report of three cases. Journal of Neurosurgery. 1977;**47**(1):96-100

[76] Brierley J, Field E. The connexions of the spinal sub-arachnoid space with the lymphatic system. Journal of Anatomy. 1948;**82**(Pt 3):153-166

[77] Elman R. Spinal arachnoid granulations with especial reference to the cerebrospinal fluid. Johns Hopkins Hospital Bulletin. 1923;**34**:99-104

[78] Hammerstad JP, Lorenzo AV, Cutler R. Iodide transport from the spinal subarachnoid fluid in the cat. American Journal of Physiology-Legacy Content. 1969;**216**(2):353-358

[79] Lorenzo A, Hammerstad J, Cutler R. Cerebrospinal fluid formation

and absorption and transport of iodide and sulfate from the spinal subarachnoid space. Journal of the Neurological Sciences. 1970;**10**(3):247-258

[80] Payner TD, Prenger E, Berger TS, Crone KR. Acquired Chiari malformations: Incidence, diagnosis, and management. Neurosurgery. 1994;**34**(3):429-434

[81] Milhorat TH, Nishikawa M, Kula RW, Dlugacz YD. Mechanisms of cerebellar tonsil herniation in patients with Chiari malformations as guide to clinical management. Acta Neurochirurgica. 2010;**152**(7): 1117-1127

[82] Tubbs RS, Oakes WJ. The Chiari malformations: A historical context. In: Shane Tubbs R, Jerry Oakes W, editors. The Chiari Malformations. New York: Springer; 2013. pp. 5-11

[83] Wilkins RH, Brody IA. The Arnold-Chiari malformation. Archives of Neurology. 1971;**25**(4):376-377

[84] Killeen A, Roguski M, Chavez A, Heilman C, Hwang S. Non-operative outcomes in Chiari I malformation patients. Journal of Clinical Neuroscience. 2015;**22**(1):133-138

[85] Nishizawa S, Yokoyama T, Yokota N, Tokuyama T, Ohta S. Incidentally identified syringomyelia associated with Chiari I malformations: Is early interventional surgery necessary? Neurosurgery. 2001;**49**(3):637-641

[86] Massimi L, Frassanito P, Bianchi F, Tamburrini G, Caldarelli M. Bony decompression vs duraplasty for Chiari I malformation: Does the eternal dilemma matter? Child's Nervous System. 2019;**35**(10):1-12

[87] Abd-El-Barr M, Groff MW. Less is more: Limiting the size of posterior fossa decompressions in Chiari I malformations. World Neurosurgery. 2014;**81**(5-6):706

[88] Lee HS, Lee S-H, Kim ES, Kim J-S, Lee J-I, Shin HJ, et al. Surgical results of arachnoid-preserving posterior fossa decompression for Chiari I malformation with associated syringomyelia. Journal of Clinical Neuroscience. 2012;**19**(4):557-560

[89] Kennedy BC, Kelly KM, Phan MQ, Bruce SS, McDowell MM, Anderson RC, et al. Outcomes after suboccipital decompression without dural opening in children with Chiari malformation type I. Journal of Neurosurgery: Pediatrics. 2015;**16**(2):150-158

[90] Navarro R, Olavarria G, Seshadri R, Gonzales-Portillo G, McLone DG, Tomita T. Surgical results of posterior fossa decompression for patients with Chiari I malformation. Child's Nervous System. 2004;**20**(5):349-356

[91] Hida K, Iwasaki Y, Koyanagi I, Sawamura Y, Abe H. Surgical indication and results of foramen magnum decompression versus syringosubarachnoid shunting for syringomyelia associated with Chiari I malformation. Neurosurgery. 1995;**37**(4):673-679

[92] Munshi I, Frim D, Stine-Reyes R, Weir BK, Hekmatpanah J, Brown F. Effects of posterior fossa decompression with and without duraplasty on Chiari malformation-associated hydromyelia. Neurosurgery. 2000;**46**(6):1384-1390

[93] Quon JL, Grant RA, DiLuna ML. Multimodal evaluation of CSF dynamics following extradural decompression for Chiari malformation type I. Journal of Neurosurgery: Spine. 2015;**22**(6):622-630

[94] Oral S, Yilmaz A, Kucuk A, Tumturk A, Menku A. Comparison of dural splitting and duraplasty in patients with Chiari type I malformation: Relationship between

tonsillo-dural distance and syrinx cavity. Turkish Neurosurgery. 2019;**29**(2):229-236

[95] Gardner WJ, Goodall RJ. The surgical treatment of Arnold-Chiari malformation in adults: An explanation of its mechanism and importance of encephalography in diagnosis. Journal of Neurosurgery. 1950;**7**(3):199-206

[96] Krieger MD, McComb JG, Levy ML. Toward a simpler surgical management of Chiari I malformation in a pediatric population. Pediatric Neurosurgery. 1999;**30**(3):113-121

[97] Logue V, Edwards MR. Syringomyelia and its surgical treatment--an analysis of 75 patients. Journal of Neurology, Neurosurgery, and Psychiatry. 1981;**44**(4):273-284

[98] Kurzbuch AR, Jayamohan J, Magdum S. Decompressive surgery for Chiari I malformation in children without dural repair: A still effective and safe procedure? Child's Nervous System. 2019;**35**(10):1-8

[99] Aghakhani N, Parker F, David P, Morar S, Lacroix C, Benoudiba F, et al. Long-term follow-up of Chiari-related syringomyelia in adults: Analysis of 157 surgically treated cases. Neurosurgery. 2009;**64**(2):308-315

[100] Alfieri A, Pinna G. Long-term results after posterior fossa decompression in syringomyelia with adult Chiari type I malformation. Journal of Neurosurgery: Spine. 2012;**17**(5):381-387

[101] Armonda RA, Citrin CM, Foley KT, Ellenbogen RG. Quantitative cine-mode magnetic resonance imaging of Chiari I malformations: An analysis of cerebrospinal fluid dynamics. Neurosurgery. 1994;**35**(2):214-224

[102] Bonney PA, Maurer AJ, Cheema AA, Duong Q, Glenn CA, Safavi-Abbasi S, et al. Clinical significance of changes in pB–C2 distance in patients with Chiari type I malformations following posterior fossa decompression: A single-institution experience. Journal of Neurosurgery: Pediatrics. 2016;**17**(3):336-342

[103] Radmanesh A, Greenberg JK, Chatterjee A, Smyth MD, Limbrick DD, Sharma A. Tonsillar pulsatility before and after surgical decompression for children with Chiari malformation type 1: An application for true fast imaging with steady state precession. Neuroradiology. 2015;**57**(4):387-393

[104] Singhal GD, Singhal S, Agrawal G, Singhal D, Arora V. Surgical experience in pediatric patients with Chiari-I malformations aged ≤ 18 years. Journal of Neurosciences in Rural Practice. 2019;**10**(1):85

[105] Zhang L, Yi Z, Duan H, Li L. A novel autologous duraplasty in situ technique for the treatment of Chiari malformation type I. Journal of Neurosurgery. 2017;**126**(1):91-97

[106] Alden TD, Ojemann JG, Park T. Surgical treatment of Chiari I malformation: Indications and approaches. Neurosurgical Focus. 2001;**11**(1):1-5

[107] Milhorat TH, Johnson WD, Miller JI, Bergland RM, Hollenberg-Sher J. Surgical treatment of syringomyelia based on magnetic resonance imaging criteria. Neurosurgery. 1992;**31**(2):231-245

[108] Ladner TR, Dewan MC, Day MA, Shannon CN, Tomycz L, Tulipan N, et al. Evaluating the relationship of the pB–C2 line to clinical outcomes in a 15-year single-center cohort of pediatric Chiari I malformation. Journal of Neurosurgery: Pediatrics. 2015;**15**(2):178-188

[109] Batzdorf U. Chiari I malformation with syringomyelia: Evaluation of

surgical therapy by magnetic resonance imaging. Journal of Neurosurgery. 1988;**68**(5):726-730

[110] Alzate JC, Kothbauer KF, Jallo GI, Epstein FJ. Treatment of Chiari type I malformation in patients with and without syringomyelia: A consecutive series of 66 cases. Neurosurgical Focus. 2001;**11**(1):1-9

[111] Stanko KM, Lee YM, Rios J, Wu A, Sobrinho GW, Weingart JD, et al. Improvement of syrinx resolution after tonsillar cautery in pediatric patients with Chiari type I malformation. Journal of Neurosurgery: Pediatrics. 2016;**17**(2):174-181

[112] Rocque BG, Oakes WJ. Surgical treatment of Chiari I malformation. Neurosurgery Clinics. 2015;**26**(4):527-531

[113] Ratre S, Yadav N, Yadav YR, Parihar VS, Bajaj J, Kher Y. Endoscopic management of Arnold-Chiari malformation type I with or without syringomyelia. Journal of Neurological Surgery Part A: Central European Neurosurgery. 2018;**79**(01):045-051

[114] Zagzoog N, Reddy KK. Use of minimally invasive tubular retractors for foramen magnum decompression of Chiari malformation: A technical note and case series. World Neurosurgery. 2019;**128**:248-253

[115] Di X, Luciano MG, Benzel EC. Acute respiratory arrest following partial suboccipital cranioplasty for cerebellar ptosis from Chiari malformation decompression: Report of 2 cases. Neurosurgical Focus. 2008;**25**(6):E12

[116] Holly LT, Batzdorf U. Management of cerebellar ptosis following craniovertebral decompression for Chiari I malformation. Journal of Neurosurgery. 2001;**94**(1):21-26

[117] Chou Y-C, Sarkar R, Osuagwu FC, Lazareff JA. Suboccipital craniotomy in the surgical treatment of Chiari I malformation. Child's Nervous System. 2009;**25**(9):1111-1114

[118] Dewaele F, Kalmar AF, Baert E, Van Haver A, Hallaert G, De Mets F, et al. The use of the trendelenburg position in the surgical treatment of extreme cerebellar slump. British Journal of Neurosurgery. 2016;**30**(1):115-119

[119] Heller JB, Lazareff J, Gabbay JS, Lam S, Kawamoto HK, Bradley JP. Posterior cranial fossa box expansion leads to resolution of symptomatic cerebellar ptosis following Chiari I malformation repair. The Journal of Craniofacial Surgery. 2007;**18**(2): 274-280

[120] Nishikawa M, Ohata K, Baba M, Terakawa Y, Hara M. Chiari I malformation associated with ventral compression and instability: One-stage posterior decompression and fusion with a new instrumentation technique. Neurosurgery. 2004;**54**(6):1430-1435

[121] Sakamoto H, Nishikawa M, Hakuba A, Yasui T, Kitano S, Nakanishi N, et al. Expansive suboccipital cranioplasty for the treatment of syringomyelia associated with Chiari malformation. Acta Neurochirurgica. 1999;**141**(9):949-961

[122] Takayasu M, Takagi T, Hara M, Anzai M. A simple technique for expansive suboccipital cranioplasty following foramen magnum decompression for the treatment of syringomyelia associated with Chiari I malformation. Neurosurgical Review. 2004;**27**(3):173-177

[123] Assina R, Meleis AM, Cohen MA, Iqbal MO, Liu JK. Titanium mesh-assisted dural tenting for an expansile suboccipital cranioplasty in the

treatment of Chiari 1 malformation. Journal of Clinical Neuroscience. 2014;**21**(9):1641-1646

[124] Oró JJ, Mueller DM. Posterior fossa decompression and reconstruction in adolescents and adults with the Chiari I malformation. Neurological Research. 2011;**33**(3):261-271

[125] Udani V, Holly LT, Chow D, Batzdorf U. Posterior fossa reconstruction using titanium plate for the treatment of cerebellar ptosis after decompression for Chiari malformation. World Neurosurgery. 2014;**81**(5-6):836-841

[126] Rahman A, Rana MS, Bhandari PB, Asif DS, Uddin ANW, Obaida ASMA, et al. "Stealth cranioplasty:" a novel endeavor for symptomatic adult Chiari I patients with syringomyelia: Technical note, appraisal, and philosophical considerations. Journal of Craniovertebral Junction and Spine. 2017;**8**(3):243

[127] Sahuquillo J, Rubio E, Poca M-A, Rovira A, Rodriguez-Baeza A, Cervera C. Posterior fossa reconstruction: A surgical technique for the treatment of Chiari I malformation and Chiari I/syringomyelia complex–preliminary results and magnetic resonance imaging quantitative assessment of hindbrain migration. Neurosurgery. 1994;**35**(5):874-885

Section 2

Imaging and Adjuvant Therapies

Chapter 5

Oncological, Vascular, and Spinal Uses of Contrast-Enhanced Ultrasound in Neurosurgery

Giuseppe Maria Della Pepa

Abstract

Contrast-enhanced ultrasound (CEUS) is a real-time, feasible technique. Both intraoperatively and bedside, it satisfies the need for serial assessment and easy performability. Initially employed in neuro-oncology, it has recently overcome this first application. The chapter aims to give a comprehensive view of its use in oncological, vascular, and spinal neurosurgery. CEUS versatility across the aforementioned areas is analyzed, underlining its complementarity to other well-settled imaging techniques. Its major oncological (both cerebral and spinal) and vascular (including aneurysms, AVMs, dAVFs, carotid plaques, and stroke) application and state of the art are discussed. The chapter is focused on reporting CEUS advantages and disadvantages, giving an insight to future perspectives and applications.

Keywords: contrast-enhanced ultrasound, CEUS, ultrasonography, brain tumors, spinal tumors, intraoperative imaging, neuro-oncology

1. Introduction

Neurosurgery is experiencing the rediscovery of intraoperative ultrasound (ioUS). In particular, growing enthusiasm was shown after the introduction of contrast-enhanced ultrasound (CEUS) in the field of neuro-oncology, following the leads of other surgeries such as thyroid and hepatic surgery. Besides this pioneering use in brain and spinal oncology, other applications including stroke, brain traumatology, vascular neurosurgery, and peripheral nerve surgery [1–9] were reported.

Those experiences in literature proved the integration of ioUS and CEUS to be a valuable tool in different neurosurgical scenarios: it provides a truly real-time, feasible, and modern intraoperative imaging technique, allowing the assessment of unexposed, hidden, anatomical, and pathological structures [10] in both traditional and emerging settings.

2. CEUS in neurosurgery: where do we stand?

Standard B-mode ultrasound has been presented since several years in many neurosurgical operating rooms: it represented de facto one of the first tools to study anatomy through unexposed, hidden, parenchymal tissues. For this reason, it is incorrect to classify ioUS/CEUS use as an innovation, being it more a rediscovery:

ioUS has been employed in neurosurgery since the 1960s [11], and it granted intraoperative imaging and navigation well before more evolved technologies, such as intraoperative CT (iCT), intraoperative MRI (iMRI), indocyanine green video angiography (ICG-VA), and navigation, were broadly available [12–15]

Nonetheless, significant limitations of ioUS as a reliable and feasible application in neurosurgery were represented by both imaging interpretation, unfamiliar to neurosurgeons, and artifacts related to manipulation. A good evidence of this is that as surgical resection advances, the ioUS image quality decreases: due to surgically induced artifacts and edema, imaging interpretation becomes challenging [1]. Moreover, all information provided by ultrasound (US) relies on echogenicity of insonated structures: no dynamic information, such as overall vascularization, is given through standard B-mode ultrasonography.

Even though the aforementioned limitations could have prevented further research, major technological advancements in the US field, such as image fusion for navigation, CEUS, and elastosonography, have been developed; new applications in their usage in neurosurgery, although on a small scale, have constantly been achieved and reported in recent years [16–20].

Being capable of highlighting tumor tissue not relying on its echogenicity but on its vascularization, CEUS has been specifically found to be a versatile innovation. Introduced in other medical branches, such as hepatic oncological surgery, the technique is feasible in both diagnostic and intraoperative settings: it allows practitioners to differentiate between benign and malignant lesions, helps in localizing the target, and controls treatment efficacies [10, 19].

On the heel of these observations, CEUS intraoperative experiences have been borrowed to neurosurgery to overcome the strains of standard B-mode US imaging.

CEUS is a harmonic imaging modality that depicts the distribution of microbubble contrast agent in tissues. Thanks to their structure, sulfur hexafluoride-filled lipidic microbubbles cannot diffuse to the interstitial space, giving a representation of the vascular district only. The degree of contrast enhancement (CE) is a consequence of the density of the capillaries, which in turn is proportional to tissue activity [19, 21].

Microbubbles are visible through a contrast-specific algorithm that permits a real-time assessment of contrast enhancement, measurement of vascularity of focal lesions during different dynamic phases, and analysis of tissue perfusion; CEUS algorithm suppresses the linear US echo, thus producing a specific representation only of the microbubbles. In other words, images are a direct representation of vascularization and become independent from tissue echogenicity. Furthermore, microbubbles, being micron-sized, are not able to extravasate from vessels and behave as a purely intravascular contrast agent, allowing to study all vascular tree districts: arterial, venous, and capillary [19, 22]. On these bases, CEUS has been introduced in neurosurgery for the intraoperative visualization of brain tumors: it is a dynamic modality which permits to visualize them according to their degree of vascularization [1, 23].

This first application has led to the following use in a variety of neurosurgical fields. As shown in the herein presented review, a consistent literature has been published describing CEUS use in settings other than cerebral neuro-oncology, including spinal oncology, vascular neurosurgery (cerebral and spinal), TBI, and pediatric and peripheral nerve surgery.

Besides their undisputed value, traditional intraoperative imaging techniques (CT scan and MRI) have several limitations, including costs, temporary stop of surgical procedure, and time wasting. These important strains make iCT and iMRI hardly repeatable during surgery [12, 24].

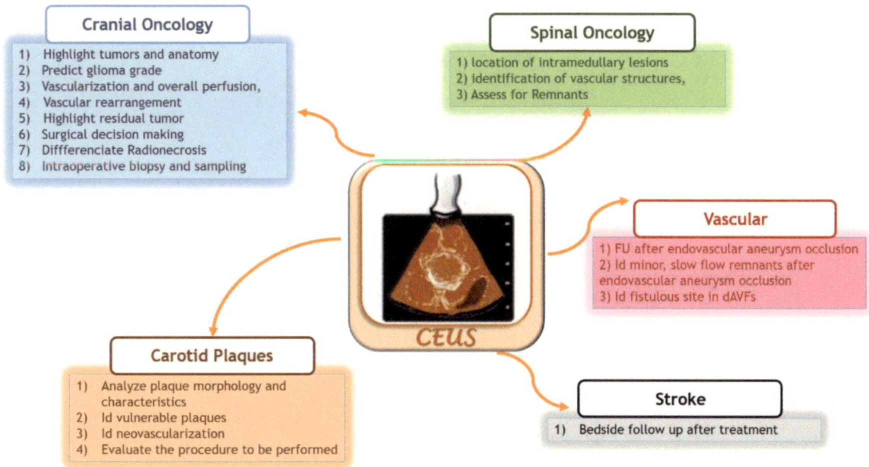

Figure 1.
Diagrammatic representation of the fields of application of CEUS in neurosurgery.

Conversely, as demonstrated by several experiences, CEUS/ioUS is a feasible intraoperative imaging technique, as it is readily repeatable, dynamic, and inexpensive and provides a truly real-time dynamic visualization of anatomical characteristics and vascular patterns in several neurosurgical settings. Assessment is rapid, can be performed any time during surgery, and is independent of brain shift [4, 8–10, 20].

Besides, microbubbles do not only allow the visualization of high-definition intraoperative images after craniotomy but, as reported later, can enhance the resolution of intracranial arteries also in transcranial studies at bedside [25–27].

Figure 1 summarizes the major fields of application of CEUS in neurosurgery.

3. Cerebral neuro-oncology

The use of CEUS during neuro-oncological procedures has been recently included in the guidelines from the European Federation of Societies for Ultrasound in Medicine and Biology (EFSUMB), representing a paradigm shift for the use of US in neurosurgery [28] (**Figure 2**).

In comparison with other imaging modes, CEUS showed itself as a rapid, practical, and cost-effective technique, suggesting additional and alternative information about brain tumor vasculature and perfusion, being B-mode limited in providing only morphological information regarding the lesion. In their seminal study, Prada et al. [29] demonstrated how, once enhanced, the tumor is highlighted and reveals other specific characteristics of both low-grade gliomas (LGGs) and high-grade gliomas (HGGs).

LGGs show a mild, dotted CE with diffuse appearance and blurred margins. Arterial feeders are usually not identifiable, microbubble transit is regular and organized, and venous drainage is diffuse through numerous capillaries and consequently not discernible. Relying not on its echogenicity but upon vascularization, CEUS proved to be particularly valuable in differentiating oncological tissue from surrounding edema, thus helping in depicting the true limits of infiltration [30, 31].

HGGs have a high CE with a more nodular, nonhomogeneous appearance and fast perfusion patterns, with a rapid CE, marked by rapid arterial phase, very fast CE peak, and chaotic transit of microbubbles within the lesion. The arterial supply

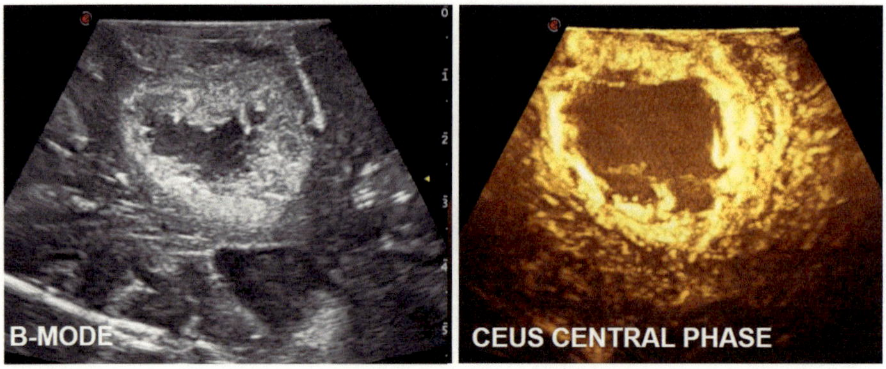

Figure 2.
B-mode CEUS evaluation of a high-grade glioma. The microbubble contrast medium allows to visualize the tumor parenchyma with its necrotic non-enhancing component. In advanced phases of resection, CEUS can be repeated to identify inadvertent residuals.

was clearly visible, showing many macrovessels within the lesion and a typical peripheral enhancement that moved toward the inner areas of the lesion. The venous phase was rapid (5–10 seconds), and the venous drainage system was diffuse, with multiple medullary veins aiming toward the periventricular zone. CEUS in HGGs is useful in differentiating solid from cystic components. In the specific case of glioblastomas (GBMs), CEUS CE is consistent in proliferating areas, and, on the contrary, no CE at all is seen in necrotic zones and surrounding brain parenchyma. Two CE patterns are identifiable in GBM: (1) heterogeneous with nodular high CE spots interspersed by low CE areas of necrosis and (2) peripheral rim CE surrounding a central core of necrosis without CE. In all cases, GBM shows a clearly demarcated border after UCA administration due to the different vascularization of the tumor and healthy brain parenchyma [29] (**Figure 3**).

Highlighting the residual tumor tissue with great accuracy and overcoming the difficulties of ultrasound interpretation caused by artifacts, edema, and surgical manipulation [10, 23, 32], CEUS has been demonstrated valuable in guiding tumor resection. In conclusion, the introduction of CEUS embodies one of the most recent innovations in HGG surgery.

Furthermore, in a series of publications, CEUS showed its capability in identifying tumor remnants after HGG surgery [10, 23, 30]. These are generally defined as nodular tissue at the edges of the surgical cavity, depicting an early and persistent enhancement, compared to the surrounding brain parenchyma. Because of artifacts due to surgical manipulation, B-mode evaluation alone can show unclear results if performed after neurosurgical resection. In the advanced phase of surgery, CEUS can fill the gap left by ioUS, guiding the surgeon also in the final survey at the end of the procedure [33]. Moreover, US is independent of brain shift, and this grants useful information to surgeons throughout the procedure also in advanced phases of resection, such as final survey at the end of the procedure.

CEUS potential in detecting inadvertent residuals proved particularly effective in a 5-ALA-guided setting [10], where the resection is built with the 5-ALA assistance, and CEUS supplementary supports the surgeon by providing information before and after resection. Incomplete resections also in a 5-ALA setting can indeed result from residual tumor covered by blood, cottonoid, or overlapping normal brain: in these scenarios it does not light up under blue light conditions and can be missed [34–37]. Moreover, in deep fields or conditions of non-orthogonal working corridors, microscope light might fail to thoroughly illuminate the surgical field, resulting in blind corners facilitating a partial removal. Thus, CEUS final survey

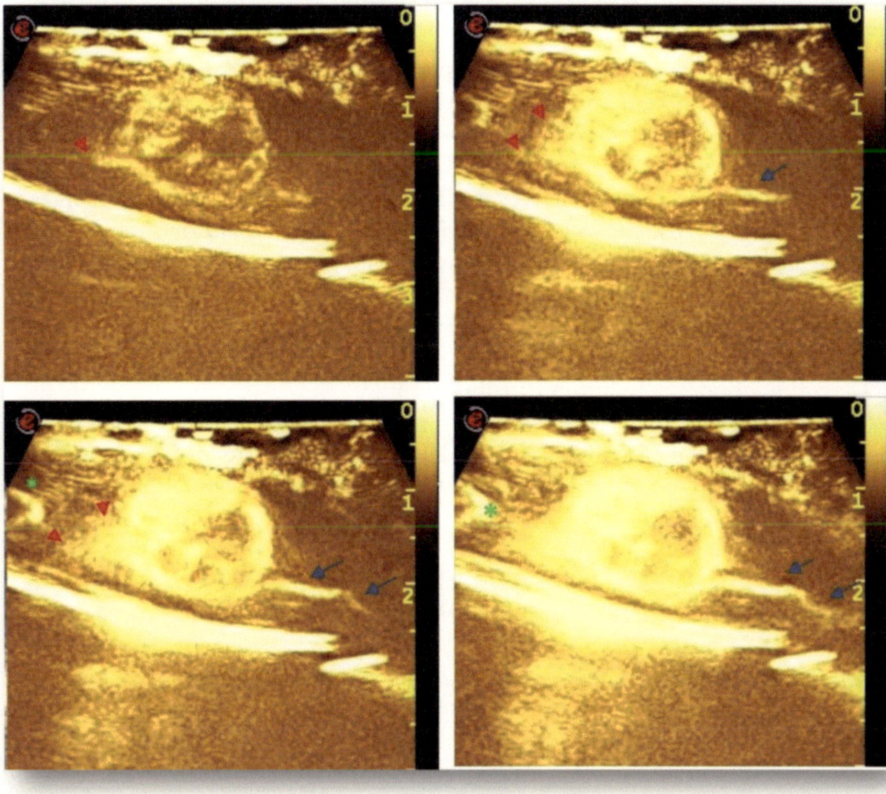

Figure 3.
CEUS visualization of lesion's vascular characteristics of a hemangiopericytoma of the cauda equina after CEUS—The exams depict the main feeders afferent to the lesion (red arrowheads) and the main venous drainage outgoing the lesion (blue arrows). The tumor is highly and rapidly enhancing after intraoperative contrast administration confirming its highly vascularized characteristics. Vessels not directly related to the tumor and belonging to conus medullaris can be identified (green asterisk).

has a role of refinement of the 5-ALA procedure by identifying sub-centimetric remnants. The two techniques approach the surgical field from a different point of view: 5-ALA fluorescence is a result of direct microscope illumination, whereas ultrasounds investigate through brain tissue, depicting also distant, unexposed, hidden cerebral or neoplastic anatomy. Indeed, they observe two different phenomena: 5-ALA is an expression of glial cell metabolism, whereas CEUS is a consequence of pathological tumor vascularization. When integrated, these complementary techniques increase the chance of identifying neoplastic residual tissue.

CEUS-assisted intraoperative imaging does not modify the overall surgical procedure, as it does not interrupt the central phase of surgery and the overall surgical strategy, is not time demanding, and does not require expensive equipment; these considerations are surely important, especially when compared with other intraoperative imaging techniques.

Also, CEUS provides other valuable information to identify vascular supply, giving further insight into the surgical strategy, facilitating vascular deafferentation and removal, and thus maximizing resection voiding neurological sequelae resulting from damaged healthy brain tissues or vessels [38].

Serious weaknesses of CEUS in vascularization assessment are angle of insonation susceptibility, low-flow veins not always visible, and small vessel overestimation due to blooming artifacts that scatter color signals nearby the vessel margins [17]. Possible limitations in the assessment of resection margin are evaluating the tumor removal degree of patients with recurrent gliomas or patients with gliomas after radiotherapy [39].

CEUS can also be compared with perfusion MRI in both preoperative and postoperative settings: US offers a morphologic representation of GBM similar to the one provided by preoperative gadolinium-enhanced T1-weighted MRI [40]. Several experiences in literature compared, instead, CEUS with pMRI in a postoperative setting [41, 42] and suggested it as a cost-effective method in evaluating changes in tumor vascularity during the follow-up period in patients with brain tumors who are undergoing radiotherapy, chemotherapy, or antiangiogenic therapy.

When combined with fusion imaging including US with MRI, CEUS has several advantages over B-mode alone [43, 44]:

1. Detection of poor sonographic visibility tumor.

2. Better recognition of the tumor and edema tissue compared with reconstructive preoperative coplanar-enhanced MRI in real time and multiplane from different angles.

3. Application by neurosurgeons who lack the expertise in US technology as an easier way to discern the structure of the brain.

4. Improved orientation and compensation for the brain shift.

Recent reports highlighted other potential applications of CEUS in cranial oncological surgery, although these experiences are still anecdotal with few cases reported. Apart from the evaluation of intraoperative resection control, CEUS has been used as biopsy guidance to correctly localize the needle and target the most representative samples for pathology [5, 45] or to guide and assess hemodynamic effects after intraoperative embolization of highly vascularized tumors such as hemangioblastomas [20, 38]. In addition, CEUS use can space from a bedside technique adding helpful information not only in noninvasive staging of tumors but also in differentiating tumor recurrence from radionecrosis as postulated by Vicenzini et al. [46] and Mattei et al. [47]; relying on microbubble diffusion through vascularization radionecrosis shows a completely different, poorer, enhancement pattern compared to HGGs.

CEUS has thus proven its utility in:

1. Highlighting tumors and their phases compared to brain parenchyma [42].

2. Characterizing glioma grade [29, 30, 48].

3. Assessing vascularization and degree of overall perfusion [29, 30].

4. Showing vascular rearrangement that takes place with tumor removal [17].

5. Highlighting residual tumor (especially feasible in a 5-ALA setting) [10, 30, 39].

6. Aiding surgical decision-making through serial imaging assessment of surgical anatomy [5, 7, 41, 42].

7. Helping in differential diagnosis of radionecrosis with neoplastic tissue due to its lack of contrast enhancement [46, 47].

8. Guiding to intraoperative biopsy and tissue sampling [5, 45]

4. Spinal tumors

Primary spinal tumors are relatively rare lesions, for which MRI represents the gold standard for diagnosis. Nevertheless, MRI may not always differentiate accurately between different types of intramedullary tumors: even if not well defined nor standardized, the role of CEUS in this surgical field appears as a problem solver. Even though a small number of cases were reported, it has proven to be a simple and relatively inexpensive technique representing a real-time dynamic procedure that can be performed during a spinal tumor surgery. Its benefits include:

1. Better characterization of the location of the intramedullary lesions [49, 50].

2. Easier identification of vascular structures, giving further insight in vascular deafferentation and then surgical removal [8, 9, 49, 50].

3. Possible combination with color Doppler to better identify the main arterial feeders and draining vessels [8, 9].

4. As for HGG surgery, CEUS helps in the identification of inadvertent remnants [8].

The important drawbacks in this setting are:

1. Possibility to analyze one portion of the lesion at the time.

2. Reduced visibility of low-flow veins and possible overestimation of small vessels due to blooming artifacts.

3. Less defined imaging due to a reduced depth of the explored surgical field compared to brain surgery [4, 8, 9]

5. Vascular applications

Providing an angiogram-like display of the parent and downstream vessel segments in high spatial resolution, CEUS might be a feasible tool for both aneurysm and arteriovenous malformation (AVM) treatment. Indeed, it could implement their intraoperative management by providing real-time imaging: this is true both in the visualization of the vascular supply before the intervention and in flow assessment at the end of the procedure [51]. Furthermore, since it allows the identification of target vessels even when covered by brain parenchyma, it could be synergistically used with ICG-VA, which relies on direct vessel visualization, in situations in which a complex approach is required [13, 52].

Focusing on aneurysms, CEUS was found particularly useful in occlusion follow-up after endovascular treatment. As opposed to a neuro-oncological setting, in which CEUS examination can be performed only after craniotomy, in the vascular setting, it can amplify vessel resolution also during transcranial examination. CEUS can selectively monitor intracranial aneurysms and detect refilling rate in aneurysms with a minor neck remnant. In the end, they suggested to perform transcranial color-coded duplex sonography (TCCS) examination with contrast enhancement at the time of initial surveillance with digital subtraction angiography (DSA) and, if findings were similar, to undertake an additional follow-up by TCCS alone until changes in aneurysm status. Transcranial examination is cost-effective, rapid, easily repeatable, and feasible compared to standard digital subtraction angiogram or angio-MRI monitoring.

To summarize, CEUS in the setting of intracranial aneurysms has the following advantages:

1. Accurate display of flow direction and velocity.

2. Increased focus and resolution, allowing detection of very low flow as often presented in coiled aneurysms.

3. Gives the possibility to be performed immediately as a control examination in the intensive care unit (ICU).

4. Produces less severe metal artifacts compared to other imaging modalities.

The main drawback underlined in both papers was the limited acoustic window in aneurysms located outside the circle of Willis, despite the introduction of contrast agent [25, 26].

In dural arteriovenous fistula (dAVF) surgery, both cranial and spinal, one of the most important steps is the correct identification of the fistulous site [53–55]. In the two reported cases [4, 56], CEUS allowed both pre- and post-ligation real-time visualization of site of the fistula and blood flow changes occurring in the spinal cord and perimedullary plexus. Not only it does encompass the limitations of Doppler imaging, which can be used simultaneously to confirm the type of flow and flow dynamics, but, as already in the case of aneurysms, it might be integrated with other imaging modalities such as fluorescence [11, 51]. However, larger series are needed to determine the significance of this tool in the obliteration of intradural spinal dAVFs [51] (**Figure 4**).

Pioneer experiences have recently been reported also in AVM surgery. Providing an angiogram-like display of the parent and downstream vessel segments in high spatial resolution, CEUS is a feasible tool for both aneurysms and AVM treatments. Indeed, it could implement their intraoperative management by providing real-time imaging: this is true both in visualization of the vascular supply before the intervention and in flow assessment at the end of the procedure. Furthermore, since it allows the identification of target vessels even when covered by the brain parenchyma, it has been proposed as a complement to standard ICG-VA.

The integration of color Doppler sonography and CEUS allows to:

1. Accurately display flow direction and velocity within the nidus and in surrounding vessels

2. Identify AVM feeders from non-AVM-related vessels

3. Evaluate the flow modifications produced into the nidus after temporary occlusion of feeders

4. Assess completeness of devascularization and eventual residual flow to the AVM

5. Assess restored venous flow into surrounding veins before dissection and isolation of the venous compartments of the malformation

Knowledge of the vascular characteristics of the AVM and the relationships of the nidus with the brain parenchyma is mandatory during these complex surgical

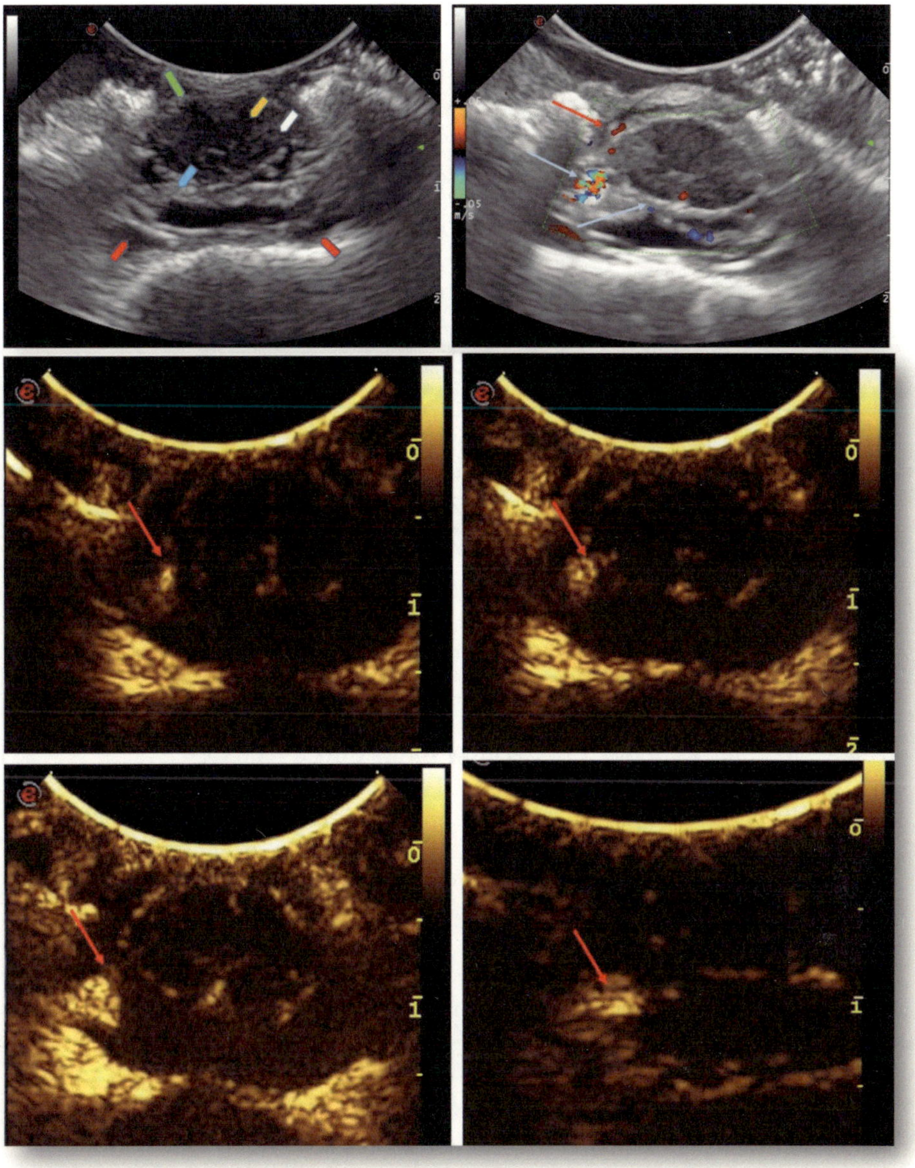

Figure 4.
B-mode and color Doppler visualization of a spinal dAVF characteristic. Epidural standard B-mode imaging showing the spinal cord anatomical proportional plan features: Green arrow, dura mater; blue arrow, peridural venous plexus; yellow arrow, spinal cord gray matter; white arrow, spinal cord white matter; red arrows, vertebral arteries. Color Doppler sonography displaying radicular artery (red arrow) and engorged peridural veins (blue arrows) with a turbulent flow. Doppler US confirms the arterialized nature of peridural plexus veins. After CEUS administration the main feeders afferent to the lesion can be observed and the main venous arterialized drainage outgoing the lesion (red arrows), thus identifying fistulous point. Peridural venous vessels not directly related to the dAVF are not visualized at this early arterial stage (arterial stage).

procedures; hence, the real-time identification of the feeding arteries and draining veins is surely valuable during surgery. Basically, the operative strategy is guided throughout the procedure by several CEUS assessments with temporary clipping of the feeding vessel, and real-time confirmation of the hemodynamic modification inside the nidus is semiquantitatively evaluated both by means of color Doppler US and CEUS. This reduces the risk of inadvertently sacrificing parenchymal non-AVM-related arterial vessels (**Figure 5**).

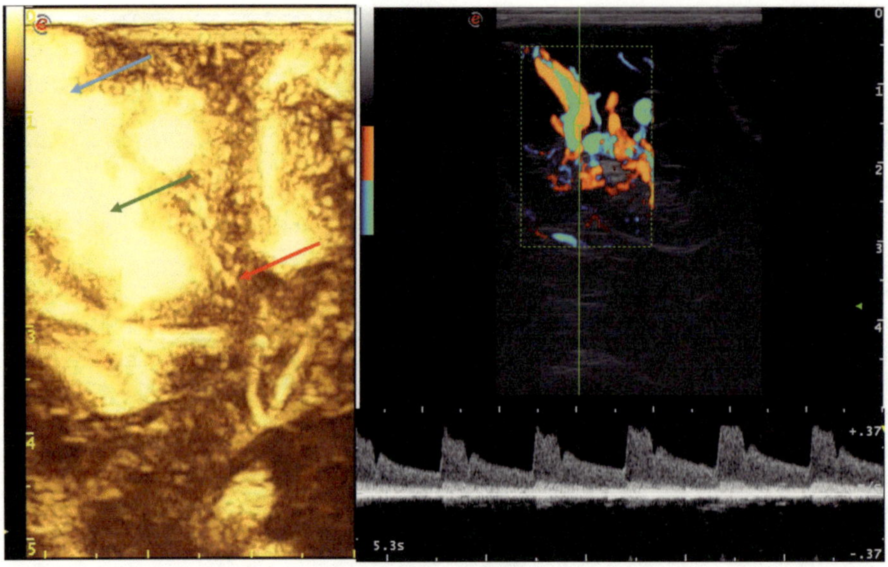

Figure 5.
CEUS and color Doppler US evaluation of an AVM, in which main arterial feeders (red arrows) can be identified, as well as the nidus (green arrow) and venous drains (green arrow). Color Doppler shows the flow direction, arterial vs. venous flow, and confirms turbulent flow within the malformation.

In advanced phases of dissection, CEUS allows the surgeon to:

a. Spatially identify in which area of the nidus residual flow is present.

b. Establish a gross estimation of the overall residual flow within the malformation (as CEUS enhancement is directly proportional to flow).

Furthermore, the restored venous flow into AVM draining veins can be reliably identified providing a final confirmation of completeness of nidal deafferentation, before the procedure is completed.

6. Stroke

An adequate supply of blood containing oxygen and nutrients is crucial for the recovery and survival of brain tissue. Monitoring of cerebral perfusion is essential in the prevention of secondary brain damage in patients with acute brain injury. CEUS has been suggested as a new method to measure cerebral perfusion in patients both with acute brain injury at the ICU and in the acute state of cerebral ischemia. The technique has a high temporal resolution which can be used at the bedside; moreover, the contrast enhancement can be used for visualization of the cerebral vasculature to overcome the restricted level of acoustic intensity. However, in this context the accuracy of CEUS for the detection of hyperperfusion has not yet been assessed.

This aligns with the idea that for patients after ischemic stroke, CEUS may serve as an additional clinical tool for the bedside evaluation of brain tissue perfusion and response to recanalization therapy, with more efforts to be made to improve its reliability [57–59]. However, when it comes to this clinical application, two key problems arise:

1. Different protocols were used by the involved research groups, and, more crucial, patients presenting with acute stroke were examined at different time windows.

2. Patients with insufficient insonation conditions were excluded in advance, and the percentage of stroke patients for which the technique could represent a consistent improvement remains questionable. Indeed, in cited studies [57–59], one of the inclusion criteria was a sufficient temporal acoustic window for conventional transcranial color-coded sonography.

As a last note, CEUS can be used as a follow-up strategy in stroke patients: it is a fast and repeatable bedside technique [3]. However, these potential advantages are undermined by (1) a small sample of studies; (2) non-validated comparison with the other imaging technique already in use in this particular area; and (3) the need for specific ecographic equipment.

7. Carotid plaques

Carotid atherosclerotic disease represents a major current health problem accounting for approximately 20% of all cases of cerebral ischemia. Risk stratification and patient management are traditionally based on the presence or absence of symptoms and the degree of stenosis, both of which have been found to correlate with the occurrence of stroke. US is the cornerstone of both screening and diagnostic approach of carotid disease, and introduction of CE has been providing promising results, leading to the publication of recommendation of use [28, 60]. An impressive number of works demonstrated CEUS is a feasible and effective tool to:

1. Analyze plaque morphology and characteristics [61]

2. Identify vulnerable plaques and detect neovascularization [62–65]

3. Perioperatively assess the procedure to be performed [66–68]

Moreover, a comparison and a proof of the relationship between CEUS and 3DT1-WI MRI plaque imaging were recently published [69]. However, on board with the purpose of this review, we decided to focus only on those works in which a prospective relationship between CEUS on carotid intraplaque neovascularization and ischemic stroke was analyzed. The grade of contrast enhancement was an independent risk factor for ischemic stroke or recurrent transitory ischemic attack. Therefore, the grade of CEUS contrast enhancement could become a predictive index of ischemic stroke, identifying those patients in need of an effective treatment. A potential source of bias coming from the exclusive selection of large plaques, a semiquantitative grading system, and a relatively small sample size are however important limitations associated with this finding.

8. Conclusions

CEUS has reached in recent years a wide utilization in various neurosurgical fields, mainly in neuro-oncological surgery. Despite its main limitations in being an operator-dependent technique and its shared drawbacks with US technology, it revealed itself as a promising tool: CEUS is comparable and complementary to traditional imaging techniques, allows for a serial assessment, is easily performable in different settings, and has a wide range of future applications yet to be explored.

Author details

Giuseppe Maria Della Pepa
Institute of Neurosurgery, Policlinico Universitario Agostino Gemelli IRCSS, Catholic University of Rome, Italy

*Address all correspondence to: giuseppemaria.dellapepa@policlinicogemelli.it

References

[1] Del Bene M et al. Advanced ultrasound imaging in glioma surgery: Beyond gray-scale B-mode. Frontiers in Oncology. 2018;**8**:576

[2] Becker A et al. Contrast-enhanced ultrasound ventriculography. Operative Neurosurgery. 2012;**71**:ons296-ons301

[3] Bilotta F et al. Contrast-enhanced ultrasound imaging in detection of changes in cerebral perfusion. Ultrasound in Medicine and Biology. 2016;**42**(11):2708-2716

[4] Della Pepa GM et al. Integration of real-time intraoperative contrast-enhanced ultrasound and color Doppler ultrasound in the surgical treatment of spinal cord Dural Arteriovenous fistulas. World Neurosurgery. 2018;**112**:138-142

[5] Arlt F et al. Intraoperative 3D contrast-enhanced ultrasound (CEUS): A prospective study of 50 patients with brain tumours. Acta Neurochirurgica. 2016;**158**(4):685-694

[6] Bailey C et al. Contrast-enhanced ultrasound and elastography imaging of the neonatal brain: A review—Ultrasound techniques for imaging of the neonatal brain. Journal of Neuroimaging. 2017;**27**(5):437-441

[7] Cheng L-G et al. Intraoperative contrast enhanced ultrasound evaluates the grade of glioma. BioMed Research International. 2016;**2016**:1-9

[8] Della Pepa GM et al. Real-time intraoperative contrast-enhanced ultrasound (CEUS) in vascularized spinal tumors: A technical note. Acta Neurochirurgica. 2018;**160**(6):1259-1263

[9] Della Pepa GM, Mattogno PP, Olivi A. Comment on the article—Real-time intraoperative contrast-enhanced ultrasound (CEUS) in vascularized spinal tumors: A technical note. Acta Neurochirurgica. 2018;**160**(9):1873-1874

[10] Della Pepa GM, Sabatino G, la Rocca G. "Enhancing vision" in high grade glioma surgery: A feasible integrated 5-ALA + CEUS protocol to improve radicality. World Neurosurgery. 2019;**129**:401-403

[11] Altieri R et al. Intra-operative ultrasound: Tips and tricks for making the most in neurosurgery. Surgical Technology International. 2018;**33**:353-360

[12] Barbagallo G et al. Intraoperative computed tomography, navigated ultrasound, 5-amino-levulinic acid fluorescence and neuromonitoring in brain tumor surgery: Overtreatment or useful tool combination? Journal of Neurosurgical Sciences. 2019. [Epub ahead of print]

[13] Marchese E et al. Application of Indocyanine green video angiography in vascular neurosurgery. Journal of Neurosurgical Sciences. 2019;**63**(6):656-660

[14] Panciani PP et al. 5-aminolevulinic acid and neuronavigation in high-grade glioma surgery: Results of a combined approach. Neurocirugía (Asturias, Spain). 2012;**23**(1):23-28

[15] Ricciardi L et al. Use of neuronavigation system for superficial vein identification: Safe and quick method to avoid intraoperative bleeding and vein closure: Technical note. World Neurosurgery. 2018;**117**:92-96

[16] Perin A et al. USim: A new device and app for case-specific, intraoperative ultrasound simulation and rehearsal in neurosurgery. A Preliminary Study. Operative Neurosurgery. 2018;**14**(5):572-578

[17] Prada F et al. Intraoperative navigated angiosonography for skull base tumor surgery. World Neurosurgery. 2015;**84**(6):1699-1707

[18] Prada F et al. Preoperative magnetic resonance and intraoperative ultrasound fusion imaging for real-time neuronavigation in brain tumor surgery. Ultraschall in der Medizin—European Journal of Ultrasound. 2014;**36**(02):174-186

[19] Prada F et al. From grey scale B-mode to elastosonography: Multimodal ultrasound imaging in meningioma surgery—Pictorial essay and literature review. BioMed Research International. 2015;**2015**:1-13

[20] Della Pepa GM et al. Erratum to 'contrast-enhanced ultrasonography and color Doppler: Guided intraoperative embolization of intracranial highly vascularized Tumors'. World Neurosurgery. 2019;**128**:547-555. World Neurosurgery. 2019;**131**:18

[21] Prada F et al. Dynamic assessment of venous anatomy and function in neurosurgery with real-time intraoperative multimodal ultrasound: Technical note. Neurosurgical Focus. 2018;**45**(1):E6

[22] Prada F et al. Intraoperative cerebral angiosonography with ultrasound contrast agents: How I do it. Acta Neurochirurgica. 2015;**157**(6):1025-1029

[23] Prada F et al. Identification of residual tumor with intraoperative contrast-enhanced ultrasound during glioblastoma resection. Neurosurgical Focus. 2016;**40**(3):E7

[24] Certo F et al. Supramarginal resection of glioblastoma: 5-ALA fluorescence, combined intraoperative strategies and correlation with survival. Journal of Neurosurgical Sciences. 2019;**63**(6):625-632

[25] Turner CL et al. Intracranial aneurysms treated with endovascular coils: Detection of recurrences using unenhanced and contrast-enhanced transcranial color-coded duplex sonography. Stroke. 2005;**36**(12):2654-2659

[26] Turner CL, Higgins JN, Kirkpatrick PJ. Assessment of transcranial color-coded duplex sonography for the surveillance of intracranial aneurysms treated with Guglielmi detachable coils. Neurosurgery. 2003;**53**(4):866-871; discussion 871-2

[27] Wendl C et al. Evaluating post-interventional occlusion grades of cerebral aneurysms with transcranial contrast-enhanced ultrasound (CEUS) using a matrix probe. Ultraschall in der Medizin—European Journal of Ultrasound. 2015;**36**(02):168-173

[28] Sidhu P et al. The EFSUMB guidelines and recommendations for the clinical practice of contrast-enhanced ultrasound (CEUS) in non-hepatic applications: Update 2017 (long version). Ultraschall in der Medizin—European Journal of Ultrasound. 2018;**39**(02):e2-e44

[29] Prada F et al. Intraoperative cerebral glioma characterization with contrast enhanced ultrasound. BioMed Research International. 2014;**2014**:1-9

[30] Prada F et al. Intraoperative contrast-enhanced ultrasound for brain tumor surgery. Neurosurgery. 2014;**74**(5):542-552

[31] Mattei L et al. Neurosurgical tools to extend tumor resection in hemispheric low-grade gliomas: Conventional and contrast enhanced ultrasonography. Child's Nervous System. 2016;**32**(10):1907-1914

[32] Trevisi G et al. Reliability of intraoperative ultrasound in detecting

tumor residual after brain diffuse glioma surgery: A systematic review and meta-analysis. Neurosurgical Review. 2019. [Epub ahead of print]

[33] Dallabona M et al. Impact of mass effect, tumor location, age, and surgery on the cognitive outcome of patients with high-grade gliomas: A longitudinal study. Neuro-Oncology Practice. 2017;**4**(4):229-240

[34] Bongetta D et al. Low-cost fluorescein detection system for high-grade glioma surgery. World Neurosurgery. 2016;**88**:54-58

[35] Raffa G et al. Multimodal surgical treatment of high-grade gliomas in the motor area: The impact of the combination of navigated transcranial magnetic stimulation and fluorescein-guided resection. World Neurosurgery. 2019. [Epub ahead of print]

[36] Raffa G et al. Surgery of malignant motor-eloquent gliomas guided by sodium-fluorescein and navigated transcranial magnetic stimulation: A novel technique to increase the maximal safe resection. Journal of Neurosurgical Sciences. 2019. [Epub ahead of print]

[37] Panciani PP et al. Fluorescence and image guided resection in high grade glioma. Clinical Neurology and Neurosurgery. 2012;**114**(1):37-41

[38] Della Pepa GM et al. CEUS and color doppler-guided intraoperative embolization of intracranial highly vascularized tumors. World Neurosurgery. 2019;**128**:547-555

[39] Yu S-Q et al. Diagnostic significance of intraoperative ultrasound contrast in evaluating the resection degree of brain glioma by transmission electron microscopic examination. Chinese Medical Journal. 2015;**128**(2):186-190

[40] Prada F et al. Contrast-enhanced MR imaging versus contrast-enhanced US: A comparison in glioblastoma surgery by using intraoperative fusion imaging. Radiology. 2017;**285**(1):242-249

[41] Harrer J et al. Comparison of perfusion harmonic imaging and perfusion MR imaging for the assessment of microvascular characteristics in brain tumors. Ultraschall in der Medizin—European Journal of Ultrasound. 2007;**29**(01):45-52

[42] Harrer JU. Second harmonic imaging: A new ultrasound technique to assess human brain tumour perfusion. Journal of Neurology, Neurosurgery and Psychiatry. 2003;**74**(3):333-342

[43] Wu DF et al. Using real-time fusion imaging constructed from contrast-enhanced ultrasonography and magnetic resonance imaging for high-grade glioma in neurosurgery. World Neurosurgery. 2019;**125**:e98-e109

[44] Wu D-F et al. The real-time ultrasonography for fusion image in glioma neurosurgery. Clinical Neurology and Neurosurgery. 2018;**175**:84-90

[45] Lekht I et al. Versatile utilization of real-time intraoperative contrast-enhanced ultrasound in cranial neurosurgery: Technical note and retrospective case series. Neurosurgical Focus. 2016;**40**(3):E6

[46] Vicenzini E et al. Semiquantitative human cerebral perfusion assessment with ultrasound in brain space-occupying lesions: Preliminary data. Journal of Ultrasound in Medicine. 2008;**27**(5):685-692

[47] Mattei L et al. Differentiating brain radionecrosis from tumour recurrence: A role for contrast-enhanced ultrasound? Acta Neurochirurgica. 2017;**159**(12):2405-2408

[48] Engelhardt M et al. Feasibility of contrast-enhanced Sonography during resection of cerebral tumours: Initial results of a prospective study. Ultrasound in Medicine and Biology. 2007;**33**(4):571-575

[49] Vetrano I et al. Intraoperative ultrasound and contrast-enhanced ultrasound (CEUS) features in a case of intradural extramedullary dorsal schwannoma mimicking an intramedullary lesion. Ultraschall in der Medizin—European Journal of Ultrasound. 2015: p. s-0034-1399669

[50] Vetrano IG et al. Discrete or diffuse intramedullary tumor? Contrast-enhanced intraoperative ultrasound in a case of intramedullary cervicothoracic hemangioblastomas mimicking a diffuse infiltrative glioma: Technical note and case report. Neurosurgical Focus. 2015;**39**(2):E17

[51] Acerbi F et al. Indocyanine green and contrast-enhanced ultrasound videoangiography: A synergistic approach for real-time verification of distal revascularization and aneurysm occlusion in a complex distal middle cerebral artery aneurysm. World Neurosurgery. 2019;**125**:277-284

[52] Scerrati A et al. Indocyanine green video-angiography in neurosurgery: A glance beyond vascular applications. Clinical Neurology and Neurosurgery. 2014;**124**:106-113

[53] Bertuccio A et al. Intracranial and spinal dural arterio-venous fistula (DAVF): A surgical series of 107 patients. Acta Neurochirurgica. Supplement. 2016;**123**:177-183

[54] Della Pepa GM et al. Angio-architectural features of high-grade intracranial dural arteriovenous fistulas: Correlation with aggressive clinical presentation and hemorrhagic risk. Neurosurgery. 2017;**81**(2):315-330

[55] Signorelli F et al. Diagnosis and management of dural arteriovenous fistulas: A 10 years single-center experience. Clinical Neurology and Neurosurgery. 2015;**128**:123-129

[56] Prada F et al. Spinal dural arteriovenous fistula: Is there a role for intraoperative contrast-enhanced ultrasound? World Neurosurgery. 2017;**100**:712.e15-712.e18

[57] Federlein J et al. Ultrasonic evaluation of pathological brain perfusion in acute stroke using second harmonic imaging. Journal of Neurology, Neurosurgery, and Psychiatry. 2000;**69**(5):616-622

[58] Seidel G et al. Perfusion harmonic imaging in acute middle cerebral artery infarction. Ultrasound in Medicine and Biology. 2003;**29**(9):1245-1251

[59] Wiesmann M et al. Parametric perfusion imaging with contrast-enhanced ultrasound in acute ischemic stroke. Stroke. 2004;**35**(2):508-513

[60] Rafailidis V et al. Contrast-enhanced ultrasound of the carotid system: A review of the current literature. Journal of Ultrasound. 2017;**20**(2):97-109

[61] Ballotta E et al. Carotid endarterectomy for symptomatic low-grade carotid stenosis. Journal of Vascular Surgery. 2014;**59**(1):25-31

[62] Hamada O et al. Contrast-enhanced ultrasonography for detecting histological carotid plaque rupture: Quantitative analysis of ulcer. International Journal of Stroke. 2016;**11**(7):791-798

[63] Amamoto T et al. Intra-plaque vessels on contrast-enhanced ultrasound sonography predict carotid plaque histology. Cerebrovascular Diseases. 2018;**46**(5-6):265-269

[64] Xiong L et al. Correlation of enhancement degree on contrast-enhanced ultrasound with histopathology of carotid plaques and serum high sensitive C-reactive protein levels in patients undergoing carotid endarterectomy. Journal of Huazhong University of Science and Technology. Medical Sciences. 2017;**37**(3):425-428

[65] Schmidt C et al. Identification of neovascularization by contrast–enhanced ultrasound to detect unstable carotid stenosis. PLoS One. 2017;**12**(4):e0175331

[66] Shao A et al. Comparison of carotid artery endarterectomy and carotid artery stenting in patients with atherosclerotic carotid stenosis. The Journal of Craniofacial Surgery. 2014;**25**(4):1441-1447

[67] Oikawa K et al. Preoperative cervical carotid artery contrast-enhanced ultrasound findings are associated with development of microembolic signals on transcranial Doppler during carotid exposure in endarterectomy. Atherosclerosis. 2017;**260**:87-93

[68] Motoyama R et al. Utility of complementary magnetic resonance plaque imaging and contrast-enhanced ultrasound to detect carotid vulnerable plaques. Journal of the American Heart Association. 2019;**8**(8). [Epub ahead of print]

[69] Shimada H et al. Evaluation of the time-dependent changes and the vulnerability of carotid plaques using contrast-enhanced carotid ultrasonography. Journal of Stroke and Cerebrovascular Diseases. 2018;**27**(2):321-325

Chapter 6

MR-Guided Laser Interstitial Thermal Therapy for Treatment of Brain Tumors

Alexa Semonche, Evan Luther, Katherine Berry, Ashish Shah, Daniel Eichberg, Long Di, Michael Kader and Michael E. Ivan

Abstract

Minimally invasive technologies for intracranial lesions are a rapidly growing area of surgical neuro-oncology. Magnetic resonance (MR)-guided laser interstitial thermal therapy (LITT) is novel adjunctive therapy for patients who are poor candidates for open surgical resection. Recent developments in modern stereotaxy, fiber optics, and MR thermography imaging have improved the safety profile of LITT, enabling its emergence as an attractive alternative adjunct therapy for intracranial lesions which are deep-seated, refractory to standard therapies, or in patients with multiple comorbidities. In this chapter, we review the technological principles underlying LITT and provide a comprehensive, up-to-date summary of the evidence regarding the indications, outcomes, and limitations of LITT for a diverse array of intracranial tumors, including dural-based lesions, metastases, gliomas, and radiation necrosis.

Keywords: LITT, laser, glioma, glioblastoma, astrocytoma, ablation

1. Introduction

1.1 LITT surgical procedure and current commercial platforms

LITT is a minimally invasive neurosurgical technique that delivers focused thermal energy from a laser light source via a fiber optic ensheathed in a catheter targeted to an intracranial lesion under stereotactic neuronavigation [1–6]. Currently, there are two Food and Drug Administration (FDA)-approved LITT platforms available for use in the United States: the Visualase Thermal Therapy System (Medtronic, Inc.; approved in 2009) and the Neuroblate Laser Ablation System (Monteris, Inc.; approved in 2007).

The Visualase and Neuroblate LITT platforms share similar components and a standardized general workflow. The patient is first induced under general anesthesia or monitored anesthesia care (MAC). The trajectory for stereotactic placement of the laser catheter is planned using standard neuronavigation technology with preoperative T1-weighted gadolinium enhanced magnetic resonance imaging (MRI) studies. The trajectory should be planned so that the catheter traverses the longest axis of the lesion without risking injury to any critical

IntechOpen

structures. Stereotactic registration of the laser catheter and trajectory planning can be performed using either a traditional headframe or frameless setup. Frameless stereotaxy requires an additional computed-tomography (CT) with fiducial markers, which is then merged with the pre-operative MRI for registration with neuronavigation.

Following stereotactic registration, a Precision Aiming Device (PAD) is aligned over the planned skull entry site using neuronavigation. A single 4 mm skin incision and burr hole is made over the entry point. The surgeon may elect to perform a concurrent needle biopsy for histopathological diagnosis. After this, a reducing cannula followed by the laser catheter is inserted through this burr hole using the PAD to ensure proper entry angle to follow the planned trajectory. Once the laser applicator probe's position is fixed using a plastic anchor bolt embedded in the skull, the patient is transferred, under anesthesia, to a MRI suite. Care is taken to prevent contamination in the operating room until T2 weighted MRI confirms the correct placement of the laser fiber. Then, near-infrared laser light (980 nm in the Visualase, system, 1064 nm in the Neuroblate system) is delivered through the fiber optic cable within the applicator probe to the target lesion. Following LITT treatment, the catheter is removed and the stab incision is closed with absorbable sutures. An example of the Visualase LITT catheter after stereotactic placement is shown in **Figure 1**.

The delivery of thermal energy to the intracranial target is controlled by several mechanisms. The fiber optic laser catheter is encased in a cooling sheath, through which cooled saline (in the Visualase system) or a $C0_2$ gas (in the Neuroblate system) is circulated. This mechanism prevents the heating of brain parenchyma along the catheter path so that thermal damage is restricted to the region surrounding the distal tip [7]. At the distal tip, the distribution of laser light to surrounding target tissue is controlled via a diffusing tip to produce a spherical zone of ablation centered at the tip. Available only in the NeuroBlate system, laser light can be delivered through a small aperture along the lateral surface of the distal catheter to provide a cone-shaped region of directional ablation.

Finally, real-time MR thermography is performed concurrently with laser ablation to generate a thermal damage estimate (TDE) heat map, i.e., a color-coded visual representation of cumulative thermal damage to structures on a T2-weighted MRI (**Figure 2**).

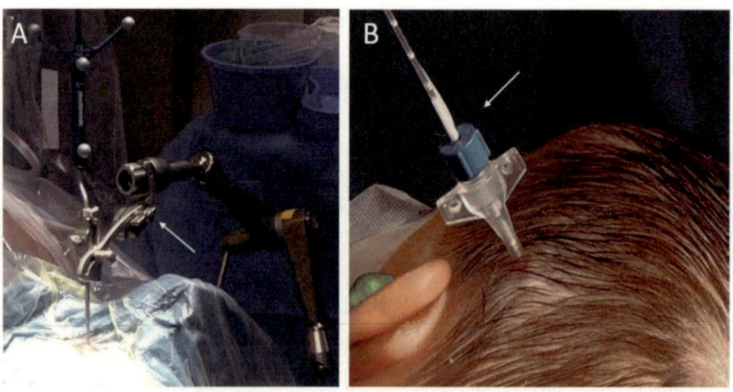

Figure 1.
(A) Intraoperative setup showing precision aiming device (PAD) (white arrow) and stealth neuronavigation wand (Medtronic, Inc.) to set laser catheter trajectory. (B) MRI-compatible laser catheter and plastic bone anchor after stereotactic PAD-assisted intracranial placement.

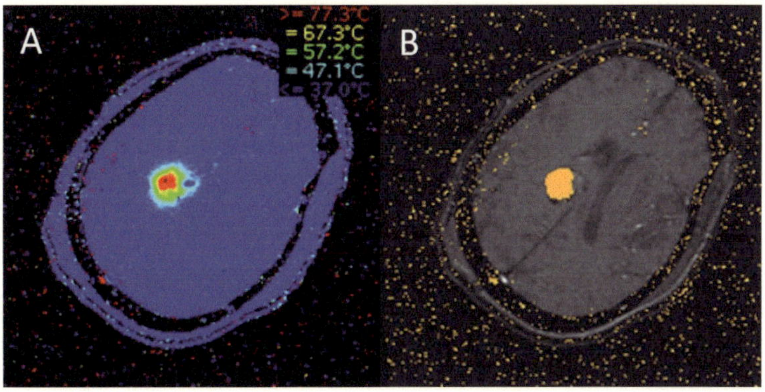

Figure 2.
(A) Real-time MR thermography provides a continuously updated heat map with concentric temperature zones. (B) Thermal damage estimate (TDE) mapping for LITT. Orange pixels estimate a zone of ablation based on a user-set threshold for sufficient ablation temperature (typically 50°C).

A computer workstation has software that allows the user to adjust laser output parameters and deliver laser energy in a series of doses until the TDE map covers the total area of the target. This is typically achieved with 10–15 W doses of laser light delivered in 30s–3 minutes intervals for a total of 10–30 minutes. The user also sets minimum and maximum temperature threshold markers on MR images defining the boundaries of the lesion. Minimum temperature markers ensure that temperatures sufficient for ablation are achieved within the target lesion volume (50–90°C), while maximum temperature thresholds ensure that off-target regions do not reach damaging temperatures [8]. Surpassing the maximum temperature threshold triggers automatic system shutoff [9]. The majority of patients have a hospital stay less than 48 hours following LITT [8–11].

Post-operative T1-weighted gadolinium enhanced MRI is typically obtained on day one following LITT, 1–3 months post-operatively, and then at longer follow-up intervals depending on clinical status. There is a typical radiographic increase in size of the ablated lesion in the acute period following LITT, peaking around 3–4 days and reaching a 45% increase in cross-sectional area corresponding to a 75% increase in volume [12, 13]. The initial increase in size seen within the first 24 hours post-op likely represents the tendency to "over-ablate" lesions and is secondary to perilesional edema that is difficult to differentiate radiographically. A significant amount of size variability is also seen in these newly ablated lesions and is attributed to multiple factors including heterogeneous gadolinium dispersion during the ablation process, heterogeneous disruption of vascular integrity, and the "extreme" variability in the amount of edema surrounding the lesion. These findings clearly lead to imaging heterogeneity and suggest that an accurate measurement of the lesion would be difficult to obtain in the first 24 hours post-LITT. Therefore, it has been suggested that MRI is more accurate at determining LITT ablation size and shape at 24 hours post-ablation rather than immediately post-LITT.

On T1-weighted gadolinium enhanced MRI, the thermal ablation zone has a thin enhancing rim with potential surrounding edema and enhancing residual blood products/protein coagulation [8]. Residual tumor remaining after subtotal ablation can be detected on this first post-operative scan. The extent of ablation can be determined by comparing volumetric analysis of the ablation zone post-operatively to the volume of the lesion on the pre-operative MRI, as described previously [14].

2. Current applications of LITT in neuro-oncology

2.1 Patient selection

LITT offers a minimally-invasive cytoreductive therapy for patients with surgically-inaccessible or treatment-refractory tumors who would likely not benefit from open surgical resection. Selection of appropriate cases for LITT is of primary concern. Over the past two decades, the first institutional experiences with LITT using MR thermography and modern stereotactic targeting were published, demonstrating both representative successes and complications associated with the procedure, including post-operative symptomatic edema, neurological deficit, and hemorrhage [4, 8, 15]. These results signaled the need to refine patient selection criteria to maximize changes of treatment success while minimizing risk of complications. From these initial studies in addition to our own institutional experiences [14, 16–18], we can summarize the following indications for LITT:

1. Anatomic location permits a reasonable expectation of an 80% ablation in order to confer a significant survival benefit [16, 19–21].

2. Lesion location is inaccessible via conventional open surgery (e.g., lesions located adjacent to deep structures such as the basal ganglia, thalamus, splenium, etc., in eloquent motor or speech areas, or near critical neurovascular structures).

3. Lesions have failed previous treatments (i.e., previous craniotomy or radiation).

4. Patients have medical comorbidities, low pre-operative functional status, or history of previous craniotomy/radiation therapy who are unable to tolerate prolonged anesthesia, blood loss, or who are at high risk of surgical morbidity and impaired wound healing.

5. Pediatrics: although cases must be carefully selected, there are currently no changes in protocol for the use of LITT in pediatric neurosurgery.

Additionally, we can summarize the following restrictions to best avoid procedural complications:

1. Functional status: patients should still have a pre-operative functional status appropriate for a minimally-invasive surgical procedure under anesthesia; in our institutional experience, patients are eligible if they have a Karnofsky Performance Score (KPS) of at least 70.

2. Lesion size: LITT should be limited to lesions with <3 cm diameter in any dimension. This size restriction stems from Jethwa et al., who reported the case of patient with a large (>3 cm) lesion treated with LITT who later underwent hemicraniectomy for medically-refractory post-ablation edema [8]. The <3 cm guideline also reduces risk of damage to critical brain regions.

3. LITT trajectory: careful precautions must be made while choosing a trajectory to avoid critical neurovascular structures. In some cases, passing through virgin white matter should take priority over creating the shorter trajectory if the shortest trajectory involves eloquent tissue.

In the following sections we review the current state of LITT for treatment for a variety of intracranial tumors.

2.2 Glioma

Recent studies have shown that greater extent of surgical resection improves progression-free and overall survival in high-grade gliomas (HGGs) [22, 23]. Although HGGs inevitably recur, some patients may not be able to undergo conventional open surgical resection due to medical comorbidities, inability to tolerate general anesthesia, or have surgically inaccessible tumor locations. In addition, risk of neurological morbidity increases with repeat craniotomy and previous radiation therapy increases risk of impaired wound healing and radiation necrosis or secondary tumor formation [24]. Up to 40% of GBM tumors are considered surgically "unresectable" based on either their location in deep or eloquent brain regions or their proximity to critical neurovascular structures [14, 25]. For these patients, laser interstitial thermal therapy (LITT) provides an alternative option for cytoreductive therapy.

The first case series reporting the use of LITT in gliomas was published in 1990 by Sugiyama et al., which described the successful total ablation of five deep-seated gliomas. This has been followed by several larger case series for both recurrent and newly-diagnosed glioblastoma multiforme (GBM) [8, 10, 11, 15, 26–30]. In these series, median recurrence-free survival ranged from 1.5 to 14.3 months and overall survival ranged from 6.9 to 16 months. These reports are consistent with estimated median survival of 14.8 and 6 months for newly-diagnosed and recurrent gliomas under standard therapy, respectively [31]. Our institutional data for deep-seated (at least 2 cm from dura) newly diagnosed gliomas further evidenced the procedural safety and efficacy in 7 patients, with a median progression-free survival of 14.3 months and 85% patients remaining alive at 14 months follow-up. As such, LITT is an emerging safe adjuvant therapy for gliomas that are considered surgically inaccessible. A recent meta-analysis reported an overall survival of nearly 14 months (range: 0.1–23 months) for patients treated with LITT and adjuvant chemoradiation, which was comparable to reported outcomes after standard treatment (gross total resection and adjuvant chemoradiation) [16, 32–34].

2.3 Dural-based lesions

Although evidence is more limited for dural-based lesions, the published studies to date support the safety and efficacy of LITT for these lesions. An initial case series by Ivan et al. reported outcomes in 5 patients with 3 recurrent low-grade meningiomas, 1 grade III malignant meningioma, and 1 solitary fibrous tumor. Ivan et al. report an average extent of ablation of 80% and a local control rate of 60% at a mean follow-up of 59.3 weeks. The procedure was well-tolerated in these patients with no complications reported [18]. Only one other case series of three patients has been reported [35]. Two patients had grade III anaplastic meningiomas while the third had a low-grade lesion. The authors report an average extent of ablation of 75% with 2 of 3 lesions recurring by 9 weeks. One patient experienced transient hemiparesis with dysarthria, which resolved.

In comparison to other reports of LITT for intracranial lesions, these studies report lower extent of ablation rates, which may be attributable to tissue consistency. In these studies, the presence of a grade III malignant meningioma complicates the picture regarding the efficacy of LITT for dural-based lesions. Nonetheless, the procedure is generally well-tolerated, justifying further investigation into its utility for these lesions.

2.4 Brain metastases

LITT is a promising adjuvant therapy for recurrent brain metastases refractory to stereotactic radiosurgery (SRS). The first case series of LITT for brain metastases was reported by Carpentier et al. [41]. A subsequent Phase I clinical trial by the same authors, published in 2011, reported 6-month local control rates of 60 and 85% for partially and fully-ablated metastatic tumors, respectively [36]. In 2016, Ali et al. identified an 80% extent of ablation threshold, below which all cases eventually recurred [37]. Similarly, Ahluwalia et al. reported a 0% recurrence rate in 100% ablated lesions [38]. A recent systematic review found that reports of median overall survival after LITT for metastases ranged from 5.8 to 19.8 months [39]. Across studies, the most commonly reported complications were temporary neurologic deficit due to unintentional thermal ablation of eloquent structures, followed by hemorrhage. Although a 1–3 day period of post-operative edema on T2 FLAIR MRI sequences frequently occurs post-ablation, this typically resolves. In four rare instances of malignant edema requiring hemicraniectomy, the lesion volumes were far greater than 3 cm in diameter [39]. These recent studies support that LITT is safe and effective in cases where 80–100% lesional ablation can be achieved.

2.5 Radiation necrosis

LITT was first described for radiation necrosis (RN) by Rahmathulla et al. [40]. In this report, a single patient presented with progressive dysphagia following radiosurgery for brain metastasis almost 2 years prior. Because the symptoms did not respond to medical management with steroids, he was treated with LITT. Following LITT, he achieved steroid independence [40]. This study was followed by larger single-center retrospective case series which reported use of LITT for radiation necrosis with initial diagnoses of glioma or metastases. In these studies <50% of patients achieved steroid freedom, and up to 20% of patients required open craniotomy for surgical resection in the months following LITT [38]. In a study of LITT for radiation necrosis or post-radiosurgery recurrent metastasis, Rao et al., reported a median progression-free survival of 37 weeks with only 2 recurrences in 15 patients [5]. The authors concluded that LITT is a safe, well-tolerated procedure for patients with radiation necrosis or metastatic recurrence.

Our institutional experience with 20 patients with biopsy-proven RN between 2015 and 2018 also supports these conclusions (unpublished data). At 1 year follow-up, 80% of patients remained recurrence free, with a median progression-free survival of 12.3 and 24.4 months overall survival. No permanent complications occurred (unpublished data).

Overall evidence supports LITT as a safe procedure for radiation necrosis that is medically refractory or surgically inaccessible. In these patients, steroid freedom as well as progression-free and overall survival are important clinical outcomes.

3. Illustrative case series

Here we present four cases of patients treated by the department of surgical neuro-oncology at the University of Miami illustrating the use of LITT for gliomas, dural-based lesions, brain metastases, and radiation necrosis.

3.1 Case 1: recurrent glioma

A 37-year-old female with previous history of left frontoparietal craniotomy and chemoradiation for high-grade glioma 2 years prior presented with progressive enhancement on surveillance MRI suggesting recurrence (**Figure 3A**). The patient was recommended LITT due to the lesion's proximity to the left motor strip. The lesion was ablated according to the following parameters:

1. Test dose at 3 W for 30 seconds to confirm location of catheter tip on MR thermography.

2. Increase in laser power to 50% maximum power for up to 3 minutes.

3. Increase in laser power at 20% maximum intervals for 30 seconds—1.5 minutes in series until maximal ablation zone is achieved (**Figure 3B**).

The patient recovered without complications. Although some residual tumor was present on postoperative imaging (**Figure 3C**), the patient remained recurrence free for 24.3 weeks with an overall survival of 1 year.

3.2 Case 2: meningioma

A 65-year-old female with previous history of craniotomy for resection of a right parafalcine meningioma and subsequent craniectomy for a wound infection

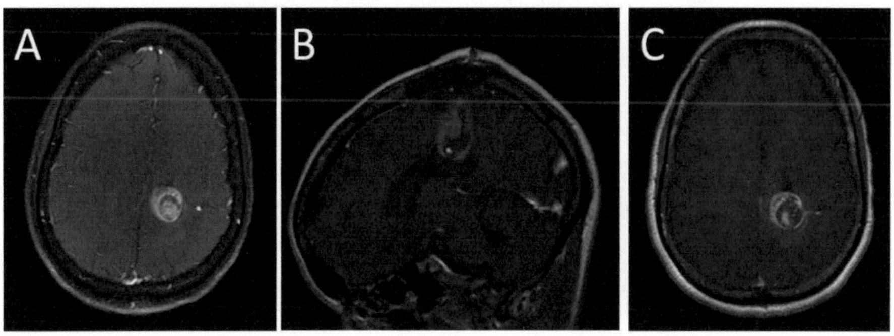

Figure 3.
(A) A 37-year-old female with periventricular ring-enhancing mass abutting the left motor strip on axial T1-weighted MRI with contrast. (B) Intraoperative sagittal MRI showing laser catheter trajectory. (C) Immediate post-operative axial T1-weighted MRI with contrast demonstrating near-total lesional ablation.

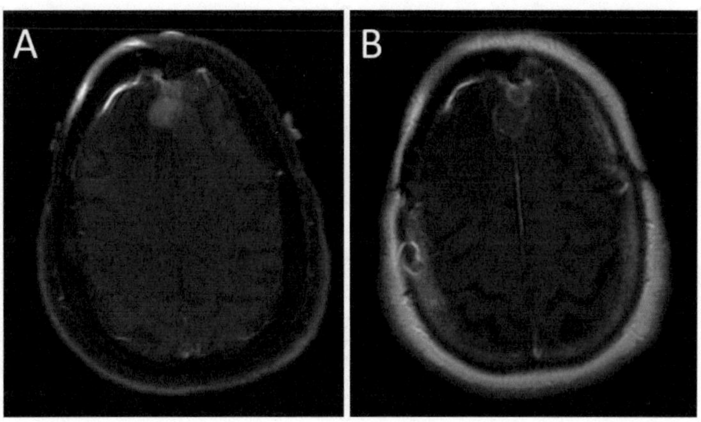

Figure 4.
(A) Pre-operative T1-weighted MRI with contrast showing recurrence of right parafalcine meningioma. (B) Post-operative T1-weighted MRI with contrast showing near-total lesional ablation.

at an outside institution presented with progressive lesion regrowth over several MRI studies (**Figure 4A**). Because of her complicated surgical history, she was recommended LITT. Postoperative MRI imaging showed 97% extent of ablation (**Figure 4B**) and the patient recovered without complications. Patient remained recurrence free until non-neurologic death 4 years later.

3.3 Case 3: metastasis

A 31-year-old female with past medial history of metastatic breast cancer previously treated with whole brain radiation and stereotactic radiation for five intracranial metastatic lesions. She presented with headaches photophobia, dizziness, and fatigue. T1-weighted gadolinium enhanced MRI showed interval growth of one lesion in the right parietal lobe. Due to her extensive previous radiation history and the proximity of the lesion to the receptive speech area of the posterior left temporal lobe, the patient was treated with LITT, achieving near-total

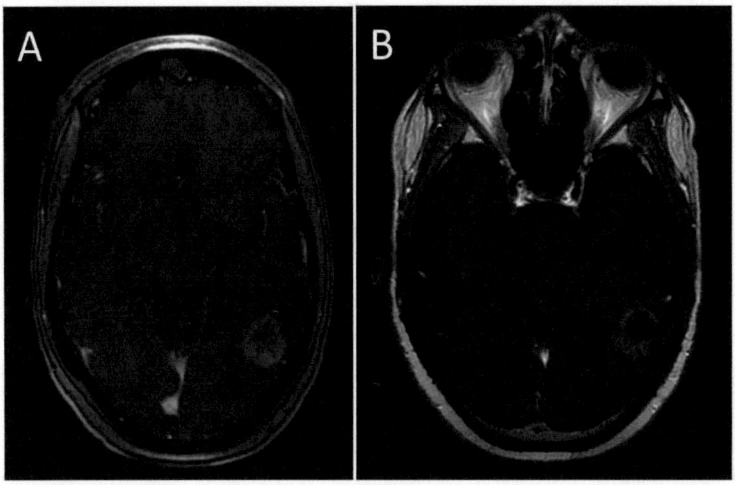

Figure 5.
(A) A 31-year-old female patient with recurrent metastatic breast cancer adjacent to the receptive speech area of the posterior temporal lobe. (B) Post-LITT procedure T1-weighted MRI shows lesional ablation.

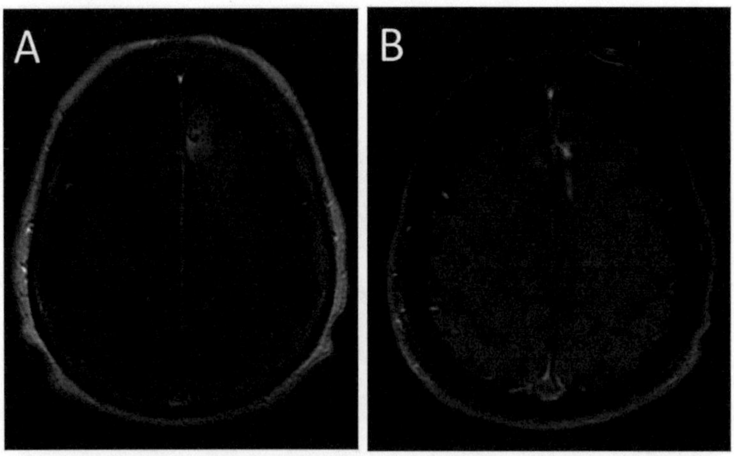

Figure 6.
(A) A 69-year-old female patient with progressive enhancement after treatment of metastatic lung adenocarcinoma. (B) Post-LITT procedure T1-weighted MRI with contrast shows successful lesion ablation.

ablation (**Figure 5B**). Patient remained recurrence free until last follow-up at 16 months post-procedure.

3.4 Case 4: radiation necrosis

A 69-year-old woman with history of metastatic lung adenocarcinoma previously treated with open surgical resection and stereotactic radiosurgery presented with asymptomatic progressive enhancement on surveillance MRI (**Figure 6A**). Because of her treatment history, the patient elected to undergo LITT. Patient recovered without complications and remained recurrence free at last follow-up, over 1 year after LITT (**Figure 6B**). Intraoperative needle biopsy performed prior to laser catheter placement confirmed diagnosis of radiation necrosis.

4. Discussion

4.1 Current role of LITT in neurosurgery

Technological advances in MR thermography and stereotactic surgery over the past two decades have facilitated the development of commercial LITT platforms. Evidence from both prospective and retrospective studies show that LITT is a safe alternative for cytoreduction in a wide variety of intracranial lesions, including metastases, radiation necrosis, dural-based lesions, and gliomas.

The advantage of LITT in treating intracranial lesions include:

1. Cytoreductive therapy in poor open-surgical candidates: a minimally invasive approach through a single burr hole reduces the risk of morbidity associated with craniotomy for surgical resection. This is especially relevant for patients who previously underwent open craniotomy or maximal radiotherapy, who are at higher risk of neurological sequelae and wound infection with repeat craniotomy [21, 24] or in patients with tumors in deep or eloquent regions of brain that would otherwise be considered surgically inaccessible.

2. Short procedure time: LITT has a shorter procedure time compared to open craniotomy. With shorter recovery times, LITT does not interrupt chemotherapy or other adjuvant therapy [10, 17].

3. Potential for repeated use: unlike stereotactic radiosurgery, LITT can be repeatedly applied and can thus be used as a salvage therapy in treatment-refractory tumors while avoiding the increased risk of secondary malignancy or radiation necrosis associated with ionizing radiation [7, 16].

Patient selection is of critical importance to ensure safe and effective use of LITT. To summarize, lesions should be <3 cm in diameter, in a region that can be accessed via a linear laser catheter trajectory without injury to critical structures and in patients who are able to tolerate a minimally-invasive surgical procedure under anesthesia. In addition, the lesion should have identifiable margins such that at least 80% of the target area can be feasibly ablated with a roughly-spherical ablation zone.

4.2 Limitations of LITT

Limitations of LITT include complications; the most common adverse events include intracranial hemorrhage and transient neurological deficit [10, 39, 41].

Intracranial hemorrhage may be secondary to laser catheter misplacement, off-target thermal ablation, or (in the case of brain metastases) an underlying patient coagulopathy [8, 39, 42]. This risk can be reduced with preoperative neuroimaging (e.g., computed tomography angiogram (CTA)) to better inform laser trajectory planning. Estimates of hemorrhage range from 0.98 to 14.2% of cases [39, 42].

Permanent neurological deficits are rare [42], but transient neurological deficits have been reported to occur in up to 35% of patients [39, 42]. Examples of commonly reported neurological deficits include weakness, hemianopsia, seizures, and dysphagia are often attributed to direct thermal injury to functional brain areas or cerebral edema. Cerebral edema is frequently observed in the immediate post-operative period following LITT, but is unlikely to cause permanent neurological deficits and may be controlled with a short course of steroids. Treatment of large (>3 cm) or use of multiple laser probes or laser trajectories is associated with a higher risk of significant cerebral edema [43].

Rare (<5% of all cases) complications include permanent neurological deficit, malignant cerebral edema requiring hemicraniectomy, infection (e.g., ventriculitis, meningitis, or brain abscess), diabetes insipidus, hyponatremia, and intracranial hypertension. There are only two recorded deaths attributed to LITT in the literature, from postoperative meningitis and intracranial hemorrhage, respectively [44].

Another limitation of LITT is that it is only appropriate for certain patients. As discussed previously, previous treatment history, baseline neurological functional status, and anticipated extent of ablation are also factors that limit use of LITT to selected patients.

4.3 Future directions

Recent studies have focused on expanding the selection criteria for LITT, for example by staging the treatment of larger (>3 cm) lesions and application to other tumors, such as pediatric tuberous sclerosis and hypothalamic hamartomas [45]. In addition, the application of computer algorithms to better predict laser ablation dynamics may further improve the procedural safety profile [46].

Another body of research is investigating the secondary effects of LITT, including blood–brain barrier (BBB) disruption, which may offer a window of opportunity for enhanced delivery of chemotherapy [47, 48]. Other studies are investigating the potential immunostimulatory effects of LITT [49, 50]. In this sense, LITT could both ablate and facilitate a future antitumor immune response [51].

Finally, future investigations will require prospective, randomized-controlled trials to evaluate the clinical outcomes of LITT compared to other salvage therapies, such as repeat craniotomy or radiosurgery.

5. Conclusion

In this chapter we reviewed the current evidence regarding safety and efficacy of LITT for four types of intracranial lesions: gliomas, metastases, dural-based lesions, and radiation necrosis. Although future randomized controlled trials are necessary to compare clinical outcomes, the evidence so far supports LITT as a safe and viable minimally-invasive approach to cytoreduction in patients with gliomas that are poor open surgical candidates.

Acknowledgements

The authors have no source of financial support to report.

Conflict of interest

Michael Ivan is a consultant for Medtronic. The other authors have no financial, personal, or institutional interests in any of the materials, devices, or drugs described in this article. Laser Ablation is only an Food and Drug Administration approved procedure for the ablation of soft tissue.

Author details

Alexa Semonche, Evan Luther, Katherine Berry, Ashish Shah, Daniel Eichberg, Long Di, Michael Kader and Michael E. Ivan*
Department of Neurological Surgery, University of Miami Miller School of Medicine, Sylvester Comprehensive Cancer Center, Miami, United States

*Address all correspondence to: mivan@med.miami.edu

References

[1] Ascher PW, Justich E, Schrottner O. A new surgical but less invasive treatment of central brain tumours preliminary report. Acta Neurochirurgica. Supplementum (Wien). 1991;**52**:78-80

[2] Bettag M, Ulrich F, Schober R, Furst G, Langen KJ, Sabel M, et al. Stereotactic laser therapy in cerebral gliomas. Acta Neurochirurgica. Supplementum (Wien). 1991;**52**:81-83

[3] McNichols RJ, Gowda A, Kangasniemi M, Bankson JA, Price RE, Hazle JD. MR thermometry-based feedback control of laser interstitial thermal therapy at 980 nm. Lasers in Surgery and Medicine. 2004;**34**(1):48-55

[4] Patel NV, Jethwa PR, Barrese JC, Hargreaves EL, Danish SF. Volumetric trends associated with MRI-guided laser-induced thermal therapy (LITT) for intracranial tumors. Lasers in Surgery and Medicine. 2013;**45**(6):362-369

[5] Rao MS, Hargreaves EL, Khan AJ, Haffty BG, Danish SF. Magnetic resonance-guided laser ablation improves local control for postradiosurgery recurrence and/or radiation necrosis. Neurosurgery. 2014;**74**(6):658-667. Discussion 67

[6] Schober R, Bettag M, Sabel M, Ulrich F, Hessel S. Fine structure of zonal changes in experimental Nd:YAG laser-induced interstitial hyperthermia. Lasers in Surgery and Medicine. 1993;**13**(2):234-241

[7] Patel NV, Mian M, Stafford RJ, Nahed BV, Willie JT, Gross RE, et al. Laser interstitial thermal therapy technology, physics of magnetic resonance imaging thermometry, and technical considerations for proper catheter placement during magnetic resonance imaging-guided laser interstitial thermal therapy. Neurosurgery. 2016;**79**(Suppl 1):S8-S16

[8] Jethwa PR, Barrese JC, Gowda A, Shetty A, Danish SF. Magnetic resonance thermometry-guided laser-induced thermal therapy for intracranial neoplasms: Initial experience. Neurosurgery. 2012;**71**(1 Suppl Operative):133-44, 144-5

[9] Medvid R, Ruiz A, Komotar RJ, Jagid JR, Ivan ME, Quencer RM, et al. Current applications of MRI-guided laser interstitial thermal therapy in the treatment of brain neoplasms and epilepsy: A radiologic and neurosurgical overview. American Journal of Neuroradiology (AJNR). 2015;**36**(11):1998-2006

[10] Carpentier A, Chauvet D, Reina V, Beccaria K, Leclerq D, McNichols RJ, et al. MR-guided laser-induced thermal therapy (LITT) for recurrent glioblastomas. Lasers in Surgery and Medicine. 2012;**44**(5):361-368

[11] Sloan AE, Ahluwalia MS, Valerio-Pascua J, Manjila S, Torchia MG, Jones SE, et al. Results of the neuroblate system first-in-humans phase I clinical trial for recurrent glioblastoma: Clinical article. Journal of Neurosurgery. 2013;**118**(6):1202-1219

[12] Nathoo N, Toms SA, Barnett GH. Metastases to the brain: Current management perspectives. Expert Review of Neurotherapeutics. 2004;**4**(4):633-640

[13] Schwabe B, Kahn T, Harth T, Ulrich F, Schwarzmaier HJ. Laser-induced thermal lesions in the human brain: Short- and long-term appearance on MRI. Journal of Computer Assisted Tomography. 1997;**21**(5):818-825

[14] Eichberg D, VanDenBerg R, Komotar RJ, Ivan ME. Quantitative

volumetric analysis following magnetic resonance-guided laser interstitial thermal ablation of cerebellar metastases. World Neurosurgery. 2018;**110**:e755-e765

[15] Schwarzmaier HJ, Eickmeyer F, von Tempelhoff W, Fiedler VU, Niehoff H, Ulrich SD, et al. MR-guided laser irradiation of recurrent glioblastomas. Journal of Magnetic Resonance Imaging. 2005;**22**(6):799-803

[16] Ivan ME, Mohammadi AM, De Deugd N, Reyes J, Rodriguez G, Shah A, et al. Laser ablation of newly diagnosed malignant gliomas: A meta-analysis. Neurosurgery. 2016;**79**(Suppl 1):S17-S23

[17] Diaz R, Ivan ME, Hanft S, Vanni S, Manzano G, Jagid J, et al. Laser interstitial thermal therapy: Lighting the way to a new treatment option in neurosurgery. Neurosurgery. 2016;**79**(Suppl 1):S3-S7

[18] Ivan ME, Diaz RJ, Berger MH, Basil GW, Osiason DA, Plate T, et al. Magnetic resonance-guided laser ablation for the treatment of recurrent Dural-based lesions: A series of five cases. World Neurosurgery. 2017;**98**:162-170

[19] Chaudhry NS, Shah AH, Ferraro N, Snelling BM, Bregy A, Madhavan K, et al. Predictors of long-term survival in patients with glioblastoma multiforme: Advancements from the last quarter century. Cancer Investigation. 2013;**31**(5):287-308

[20] Oppenlander ME, Wolf AB, Snyder LA, Bina R, Wilson JR, Coons SW, et al. An extent of resection threshold for recurrent glioblastoma and its risk for neurological morbidity. Journal of Neurosurgery. 2014;**120**(4):846-853

[21] Laws ER, Parney IF, Huang W, Anderson F, Morris AM, Asher A, et al. Survival following surgery and prognostic factors for recently diagnosed malignant glioma: Data from the glioma outcomes project. Journal of Neurosurgery. 2003;**99**(3):467-473

[22] Brown TJ, Brennan MC, Li M, Church EW, Brandmeir NJ, Rakszawski KL, et al. Association of the extent of resection with survival in glioblastoma: A systematic review and meta-analysis. JAMA Oncology. 2016;**2**(11):1460-1469

[23] Sanai N, Polley MY, McDermott MW, Parsa AT, Berger MS. An extent of resection threshold for newly diagnosed glioblastomas. Journal of Neurosurgery. 2011;**115**(1):3-8

[24] Chang SM, Parney IF, McDermott M, Barker FG, Schmidt MH, Huang W, et al. Perioperative complications and neurological outcomes of first and second craniotomies among patients enrolled in the glioma outcome project. Journal of Neurosurgery. 2003;**98**(6):1175-1181

[25] Fazeny-Dorner B, Wenzel C, Veitl M, Piribauer M, Rossler K, Dieckmann K, et al. Survival and prognostic factors of patients with unresectable glioblastoma multiforme. Anti-Cancer Drugs. 2003;**14**(4):305-312

[26] Schwarzmaier HJ, Eickmeyer F, von Tempelhoff W, Fiedler VU, Niehoff H, Ulrich SD, et al. MR-guided laser-induced interstitial thermotherapy of recurrent glioblastoma multiforme: Preliminary results in 16 patients. European Journal of Radiology. 2006;**59**(2):208-215

[27] Hawasli AH, Bagade S, Shimony JS, Miller-Thomas M, Leuthardt EC. Magnetic resonance imaging-guided focused laser interstitial thermal therapy for intracranial lesions: Single-institution series. Neurosurgery. 2013;**73**(6):1007-1017

[28] Mohammadi AM, Schroeder JL. Laser interstitial thermal therapy

in treatment of brain tumors—The neuroblate system. Expert Review of Medical Devices. 2014;**11**(2):109-119

[29] Kamath AA, Friedman DD, Akbari SHA, Kim AH, Tao Y, Luo J, et al. Glioblastoma treated with magnetic resonance imaging-guided laser interstitial thermal therapy: Safety, efficacy, and outcomes. Neurosurgery. 2019;**84**(4):836-843

[30] Shah AH, Burks JD, Buttrick SS, Debs L, Ivan ME, Komotar RJ. Laser interstitial thermal therapy as a primary treatment for deep inaccessible gliomas. Neurosurgery. 2019;**84**(3):768-777

[31] Stupp R, Mason WP, van den Bent MJ, Weller M, Fisher B, Taphoorn MJ, et al. Radiotherapy plus concomitant and adjuvant temozolomide for glioblastoma. The New England Journal of Medicine. 2005;**352**(10):987-996

[32] Stupp R, Hegi ME, Mason WP, van den Bent MJ, Taphoorn MJ, Janzer RC, et al. Effects of radiotherapy with concomitant and adjuvant temozolomide versus radiotherapy alone on survival in glioblastoma in a randomised phase III study: 5-year analysis of the EORTC-NCIC trial. The Lancet Oncology. 2009;**10**(5):459-466

[33] Allahdini F, Amirjamshidi A, Reza-Zarei M, Abdollahi M. Evaluating the prognostic factors effective on the outcome of patients with glioblastoma multiformis: Does maximal resection of the tumor lengthen the median survival? World Neurosurgery. 2010;**73**(2):128-134. Discussion e16

[34] Lacroix M, Abi-Said D, Fourney DR, Gokaslan ZL, Shi W, DeMonte F, et al. A multivariate analysis of 416 patients with glioblastoma multiforme: Prognosis, extent of resection, and survival. Journal of Neurosurgery. 2001;**95**(2):190-198

[35] Rammo R, Scarpace L, Nagaraja T, Lee I. MR-guided laser interstitial thermal therapy in the treatment of recurrent intracranial meningiomas. Lasers in Surgery and Medicine. 2019;**51**(3):245-250

[36] Carpentier A, McNichols RJ, Stafford RJ, Guichard JP, Reizine D, Delaloge S, et al. Laser thermal therapy: Real-time MRI-guided and computer-controlled procedures for metastatic brain tumors. Lasers in Surgery and Medicine. 2011;**43**(10):943-950

[37] Ali MA, Carroll KT, Rennert RC, Hamelin T, Chang L, Lemkuil BP, et al. Stereotactic laser ablation as treatment for brain metastases that recur after stereotactic radiosurgery: A multiinstitutional experience. Neurosurgical Focus. 2016;**41**(4):E11

[38] Ahluwalia M, Barnett GH, Deng D, Tatter SB, Laxton AW, Mohammadi AM, et al. Laser ablation after stereotactic radiosurgery: A multicenter prospective study in patients with metastatic brain tumors and radiation necrosis. Journal of Neurosurgery. 2018;**130**(3):804-811

[39] Alattar AA, Bartek J Jr, Chiang VL, Mohammadi AM, Barnett GH, Sloan A, et al. Stereotactic laser ablation as treatment for brain metastases recurring after stereotactic radiosurgery: A systematic literature review. World Neurosurgery. 2019;S1878-8750(19)31195-7

[40] Rahmathulla G, Recinos PF, Valerio JE, Chao S, Barnett GH. Laser interstitial thermal therapy for focal cerebral radiation necrosis: A case report and literature review. Stereotactic and Functional Neurosurgery. 2012;**90**(3):192-200

[41] Carpentier A, McNichols RJ, Stafford RJ, Itzcovitz J, Guichard JP, Reizine D, et al. Real-time magnetic resonance-guided laser thermal therapy for focal metastatic brain

tumors. Neurosurgery. 2008;**63**(Suppl 1):ONS21-ONS28. Discussion ONS8-9

[42] Pruitt R, Gamble A, Black K, Schulder M, Mehta AD. Complication avoidance in laser interstitial thermal therapy: Lessons learned. Journal of Neurosurgery. 2017;**126**(4):1238-1245

[43] Ashraf O, Patel NV, Hanft S, Danish SF. Laser-induced thermal therapy in neuro-oncology: A review. World Neurosurgery. 2018;**112**:166-177

[44] Mohammadi AM, Hawasli AH, Rodriguez A, Schroeder JL, Laxton AW, Elson P, et al. The role of laser interstitial thermal therapy in enhancing progression-free survival of difficult-to-access high-grade gliomas: A multicenter study. Cancer Medicine. 2014;**3**(4):971-979

[45] Xu DS, Chen T, Hlubek RJ, Bristol RE, Smith KA, Ponce FA, et al. Magnetic resonance imaging-guided laser interstitial thermal therapy for the treatment of hypothalamic hamartomas: A retrospective review. Neurosurgery. 2018;**83**(6):1183-1192

[46] Jermakowicz WJ, Mahavadi AK, Cajigas I, Dan L, Guerra S, Farooq G, et al. Predictive modeling of brain tumor laser ablation dynamics. Journal of Neuro-Oncology. 2019;**144**(1):193-203

[47] Sabel M, Rommel F, Kondakci M, Gorol M, Willers R, Bilzer T. Locoregional opening of the rodent blood-brain barrier for paclitaxel using Nd:YAG laser-induced thermo therapy: A new concept of adjuvant glioma therapy? Lasers in Surgery and Medicine. 2003;**33**(2):75-80

[48] Leuthardt EC, Duan C, Kim MJ, Campian JL, Kim AH, Miller-Thomas MM, et al. Hyperthermic laser ablation of recurrent glioblastoma leads to temporary disruption of the peritumoral blood brain barrier. PLoS One. 2016;**11**(2):e0148613

[49] Vogl TJ, Straub R, Eichler K, Woitaschek D, Mack MG. Malignant liver tumors treated with MR imaging-guided laser-induced thermotherapy: Experience with complications in 899 patients (2,520 lesions). Radiology. 2002;**225**(2):367-377

[50] Ivarsson K, Myllymaki L, Jansner K, Stenram U, Tranberg KG. Resistance to tumour challenge after tumour laser thermotherapy is associated with a cellular immune response. British Journal of Cancer. 2005;**93**(4):435-440

[51] Axelsson A, Pantaleone C, Astrom S. Initial findings of immunostimulating interstitial laser thermotherapy of solid tumors. Journal for Clinical Studies. 2017;**9**:28-31

Chapter 7

Immunotherapy for Glioblastomas

Wan-Ming Hu, Frank Y. Shan, Sanjib Mukherjee, Danijela Levacic and Jason H. Huang

Abstract

Glioblastoma (GBM), a WHO grade IV brain tumor, is an aggressive tumor with poor prognosis; even with current standard care of triple therapy, consisting of surgical resection, chemo and radiation therapy, the patients' median survival time is only approximately 15 months. Recent practice shows that immunotherapy made some progress in some other solid tumors, like melanoma or non-small cell lung cancer. This chapter is going to review some advances in immunotherapy for GBM.

Keywords: glioblastoma (GBM), Blood-brain barrier (BBB), immunotherapy, epidermal growth factor receptor variant III (EGFRvIII), AMG 595 monoclonal antibody, vaccine, rindopepimut, T cells, PD-1 and PDL-1, overall survival (OS), immune checkpoint molecules

1. Introduction

Glioblastoma (GBM), a World Health Organization (WHO) designed grade IV tumor, is an aggressive and most lethal form of brain tumor with extremely poor prognosis. Although there exists a standard triple therapy (surgical, chemo and radiation), the average survival time for patients with GBM is less than 2 years. Due to the presence of blood-brain barrier (BBB), a naturally made special structure of the vascular wall inside brain parenchyma, it allows only smaller molecules get through the BBB into brain parenchyma, which makes it even more difficult for the chemotherapeutic agent to reach the target tumor cells. In addition, due to the infiltration nature of this tumor, surgical resection with GTR (gross total resection) without damage the brain function is almost impossible to archive. Radiation therapy may produce some partial control of the tumor; at the same time, it not only induces radiation necrosis but also causes additional mutation of the tumor. On the other hand, in contrast to mutations of many other solid tumors from other organ systems, most glioma-associated mutations offer slightly better prognosis for the patients, making the target therapy to those mutations less significant and less important. As mentioned above, it is vitally important and necessary to develop a minimally invasive and greatly effective method for treating the glioblastoma. In this regard, novel GBM treatments including immunotherapy are being investigated [1]. Key challenges in glioma-specific immunotherapy as with many other cancers are the limited immunogenicity of the cancer cells and the immunosuppressive environment of the tumor. Although specific antigens have been identified in several cancers, brain tumors, such as GBM, are considered poorly immunogenic [1]. In addition, the tumor's heterogeneity and its consistent mutations may contribute further to its poor immunogenicity [1].

Immunotherapy has garnered increasing support in recent years as a treatment for brain tumors. The immune system has a tremendous capacity for targeting and eliminating tumor cells while sparing normal tissues. Following decades of preclinical development and success in other solid and blood-borne neoplasms, many immunotherapies are now being investigated in patients with GBM. Immunotherapeutic classes currently under investigation in patients with GBM include various vaccination strategies, adoptive T-cell immunotherapy, immune checkpoint blockage, monoclonal antibodies, and cytokine therapy. Trails include patients with either primary or recurrent GBM.

2. Vaccine therapy

2.1 Adoptive T-cell immunotherapy (ALT)

Over the past decade, the FDA has approved emerging immunotherapies for a variety of cancers [2]. At present, many studies have proven that the brain is no longer an immune-exempt organ, and there are many interactions between tumors and the brain immune system [3, 4]. The fully functional T-cell bank plays an important part in maintaining immune surveillance and initiating antitumor immune responses. However, glioblastoma (GBM) is particularly good at destroying antitumor immunity and causing severe T-cell dysfunction. In GBM patients, both local and systemic immunosuppressive disorders impair any possible antitumor response. Woroniecka et al. [5] have analyzed and summarized the categories and molecular mechanisms of T-cell dysfunction in GBMs, including senescence, tolerance, anergy, exhaustion, and ignorance.

Adoptive T-cell therapy for brain tumors has received increasing attention as a breakthrough emerging therapy. Adoptive T-cell therapy refers to engineering specific T cells to target the tumor cells and recognize tumor-specific antigens, and eventually cause tumor cells to die through the immune response. Because T-cell immune response is strong and specific, it can distinguish tumor tissue from healthy tissue, and can target malignant cells to prevent distant metastasis, and T cells can proliferate to maintain therapeutic effect. Currently, T-cell immunotherapy includes three types of tumor infiltrating lymphocytes (TIL), T-cell receptor (TCR), and chimeric antigen receptor (CAR). Among them, CAR T-cell therapy is the only therapy that has made significant progress in clinical application. Chimeric antigen receptor T (CAR T) cell therapy refers to using the patient's own T lymphocytes, which have been re-engineered, loaded with receptors and co-stimulatory molecules that recognize tumor antigens, and expanded into the patient's body after in vitro expansion to identify and attack their own tumor cell. GBM cells can express a variety of antigens, such as human epidermal growth factor receptor 2 (HER2), interleukin 13 receptor subunit α-2 (IL13Rα2), ephrin-A2 (EphA2), and epidermal growth factor receptor variant III (EGFRvIII), which have been successfully targeted using chimeric antigen receptors T cells (CARs-T) in preclinical models [6].

Studies have shown that CAR T cells targeting EGFRvIII play a role in the treatment of GBM, and multiple trials are ongoing or under preparation. A Phase I study involving 10 patients with relapsed GBM demonstrates the safety and feasibility of EGFRvIII CAR T-cell therapy [7]. IL13Rα2-CARsT cells can produce cytokines, including interferon γ (IFNγ) and tumor necrosis factor-α (TNF-α), and display cytolytic activity by generating a pro-inflammatory microenvironment in mice bearing gliomas. Phase I trials (NCT00730613) for recurrent GBM have been completed and promising results have been shown [8]. Another IL13Ra2-targeted CAR

T-cell therapy for patients with recurrent GBM has also shown significant effects [1–7]. Ahmed and colleagues reported a Phase I study involving 17 HER2 + GBM patients treated with HER2-specific CAR-modified virus-specific T cells, which achieved safety, feasibility, and anti-GBM activity endpoint [9].

Although CAR T cells have high therapeutic potential, complex GBM biological characteristics and tumor microenvironment make CAR T-cell therapy also face challenges.

CAR T cells cannot target intracellular proteins, and tumors may shed their targets and escape treatment. There may also be insufficient proliferation of T cells, resulting in treatment that is not durable. Some researchers are engineering and modifying T cells to improve their antitumor efficacy. Interleukin 12 is an effective pro-inflammatory cytokine. Yeku designed a CAR T cell that carries and expresses IL-12, and proved that the CAR T cell has enhanced proliferation ability, decreased apoptosis, and increased cells toxicity, thereby enhancing antitumor efficacy in ovarian peritoneal cancer [10]. Kevin Bielamowicz et al. created trivalent T cells with three specific CAR molecules (trivalent CAR T cells) to overcome the patient's antigenic variability in glioblastoma. Compared with monovalent and bivalent CAR T cells, trivalent CAR T cells mediate powerful immune synapses by forming more microtubule tissue centers between CAR T cells and tumor targets, and show stronger cytotoxicity according to each patient [6].

In the future, with the continuous deepening of research, adoptive T-cell strategies will definitely open up a bright path for GBM immunotherapy.

ALT therapy has now evolved to leverage advances in gene engineering and retroviral delivery. Patient-derived T cells can be engineered with antigen-specific T-cell receptors (TCRs) or tumor-specific chimeric antigen receptors (CARs) to confer target recognition independent of and in addition to naturally occurring TCRs. The best studied of these T-cell modifications are CARs. CARs are synthetic receptors that couple the single-chain Fv fragment of a monoclonal antibody with various T-cell signaling molecules, thus endowing T cells with the antigen-specific recognition of the humoral compartment, the intracellular signaling required for cytotoxicity, and the co-stimulation necessary for sustained activity. As such, CAR T cells recognize target antigens without a need for MHC peptide presentation, circumventing one major mechanism of tumor immune escape-MHC downregulation. CAR T-cell therapy has demonstrated promising results and FDA approval for hematological malignancy is expected shortly [11].

Clinically, adoptive T-cell therapy has demonstrated its effectiveness with CAR-based treatment for CD19C B-cell malignancies. A clinical trial for 11 recurrent GBM patients has demonstrated infusions of autologous adoptively transferred human cytomegalovirus (CMV)-specific T cells increased OS to > 57 weeks, with four patients maintaining no progression throughout the study period [12].

2.2 Peptide vaccine

Peptide vaccination concerns generation of vaccine based on peptide sequences representing a tumor antigen-specific target. Peptide vaccinations offer the advantage of high specificity and ease of antigen generation. Limitations include poor immunogenicity of peptide [1].

Rindopepimut (CDX-110) is a 14mer amino acid peptide that spans the EGFRvIII mutation site conjugated with keyhole limpet hemocyanin (KLH). In a small single-arm Phase II multicenter trail, 18 patients with newly diagnosed GBM completing standard of care therapy were vaccinated with rindopepimut combined with granulocyte-macrophage colony-stimulating factor (GM-CSF) resulting in a median OS of 26 months [4]. Overall, this vaccine was well tolerated with minimal toxicity.

Another randomized Phase II trial including 65 newly diagnosed EGFRvIII-positive patients with GBM was undertaken. Patients again received rindopepimut combined with GM-CSF following tumor resection and TMZ chemoradiation. The median OS was 24.6 months. Randomized Phase III clinical trial currently underway and initial Phase III data showed increased progression-free survival (PFS) and OS from point of diagnosis [1].

3. Monoclonal antibodies to EGFRvIII

The epidermal growth factor receptor (EGFR) gene expression is associated with a malignant phenotype in multiple cancers, like colon cancer, non-small cell lung cancer, head and neck squamous cell carcinoma, and GBM [13].

The EGFR gene amplification has been reported to be the most common genetic alteration in primary GBMs (40–70%) [13]. In approximately about 50–60% of GBMs with EGFR overexpressed, there is a specific type of EGFR gene variant generally called as EGFR variant III (EGFRvIII) [14]. EGFRvIII is the most common result of gene rearrangement after EGFR gene amplification [15–17]. Histone modification of gene enhancer on chromosome 7p12 leads to EGFRvIII formation [18]. Juxtaposition of EGFR exon 1 and 8 forms a novel glycine residue between these two exons. Deletion of EGFR exon 2–7 yields a truncated transmembrane protein receptor that lacks the extracellular ligand-binding domain but retains the constitutional tyrosine kinase activity that stimulates malignant growth [19, 20]. At present, there is no evidence of EGFRvIII expression in wild type human tissues [17, 21–25]. Thus, EGFRvIII serves as a unique tumor-specific antigen and is a candidate for targeted therapy [26]. EGFRvIII can show ligand-independent activity and continuously activate downstream signaling pathway [27, 28], which promotes proliferation, reduces apoptosis, enhances tumor cell xenograft ability, and increases angiogenesis and invasion [22, 27, 29–31].

According to current research, antibodies that target EGFRvIII for the treatment of gliomas include ABT-414 and AMG-595.

Depatuxizumab mafodotin (depatux-m, ABT-414) is a tumor-specific selection antibody drug conjugate (ADC) composed of an anti-EGFR antibody ABT-806 and a potent microtubule inhibitor (MMAF). Studies by Philips et al. have shown that ABT-414 can selectively kill the tumor cells with EGFRwt or EGFRvIII overexpressed tumor in vivo xenograft models and in vitro. ABT-414 combined with radiotherapy and chemotherapy can significantly inhibit tumor growth in vivo [32]. At present, the clinical trials for the treatment of glioma with ABT-414 mainly include NCT02343406, NCT02573324, NCT02590263, and NCT01800695.

AMG 595 is an antibody-drug conjugate comprising a fully humanized, anti-EGFRvIII monoclonal antibody linked to the maytansinoid DM1, a semisynthetic derivative of maytansine. AMG595 binds to EGFRvIII but not native EGFR; after binding, the AMG595-EGFRvIII complex is internalized via the lysosomal pathway, leading to the release of DM1 and mitotic arrest and potent growth inhibition [13]. AMG 595 exhibited favorable pharmacokinetics and is a unique therapy with possible benefit for some patients with EGFRvIII-mutated GBM with limited therapeutic options [26].

4. Immune checkpoint blockade

As early as 1863, Rudolf Virchow reported the inflammatory infiltration in tumor tissues and proposed an important connection between cancer and the immune system [33]. In the following researches, the concept of "immune checkpoint molecules" was proposed. One of the important physiological functions of the immune checkpoint molecule is to keep the activation of the immune system within the normal range. Dysfunction of immunological checkpoint molecules can lead to immune evasion in many human tumors. Nowadays, immune checkpoint therapies are attracting a lot of attention from scientists who are devoted to cancer treatment.

It has been recognized that coinhibitory receptors on T cells play an essential role in attenuating the strength and duration of T cell-mediated immune responses. These inhibitory receptors are referred to as immune checkpoint molecules, which are responsible for maintaining self-tolerance and preventing autoimmune reactions [34]. To date, the two most intensely investigated coinhibitory molecules are CTLA-4 (that acts early in T-cell activation) and PD1 (that blocks T cell at late stages of the immune response). It has been demonstrated that blockade of CTL4 and PD1 could induce tumor regression and promote long-term survival in mouse glioma models [34].

Among a lot of immune checkpoint molecules, the membrane-bound molecules programmed death 1 (PD-1) and its ligand PD-L1 (PD-1/PD-L1) are the two most popular markers.

4.1 PD-1 and PD-L1

The programmed cell death ligand 1 (PD-L1) protein belongs to the B7 family, and is widely expressed in almost all tumor cells as well as many normal cells. The combination of PD-L1 and PD-1 provides a strong inhibitory signal that inhibits the proliferation, activation, and infiltration of cytotoxic T lymphocytes (CTLs) [35, 36], thereby mediating the immunosuppressive effects of tumors. This is considered to be the major negative regulatory mechanism of CTLs in the cancer microenvironment. More importantly, in addition to binding to PD-1, PD-L1 can also bind to other co-stimulatory molecules such as CD28, CD80, and CTLA-4 in cancer cells [37], which indicates that PD-L1 can mediate a broader and more complex immune regulation mechanism. Therefore, it is important to analyze the expression and cell distribution of PD-L1 in GBM tissues.

Glioblastoma (GBM) creates immune evasion and suppression, thereby evading the body's immune system and promoting tumor growth. Despite standard management composed of the maximal surgical resection with the combination of radiation therapy and chemotherapy, the median survival time of GBM patients is only 12–15 months after diagnosis [38]. At present, it is found that immunological checkpoint proteins can be blocked by related checkpoint inhibitors, thus becoming a viable target for tumor therapy. Therefore, it is very meaningful to explore new immunotherapy to counteract the immunosuppressive effects in GBM, and necessary to explore new immunotherapy to counteract the immunosuppressive effects in GBM.

4.2 Expression and cell distribution of PD-L1 in human glioma tissues

The PD-1 ligand, PD-L1 (also known has B7-H1), has been observed to be expressed in GBMs and GBM-associated macrophages, but the positivity rate in GBMs is controversial and highly variable, probably due to the selections of different antibodies by those researches [34, 39, 40]. Berghoff et al. [41] used a non-commercial anti-PD-L1 antibody, 5H1, showed membranous PD-L1 expression in 37.6% of newly diagnosed and 16.7% of recurrent GBMs, and diffuse/fibrillary PD-L1 expression in 84.4% of newly diagnosed and 72.2% of recurrent GBMs. However, in a study with 1035 GBM specimens using SP142 antibody, the positive rate of PD-L1 was only

19% [42]. Our own data, using the same standard in NSCLC (cutoff value was ≥1% of tumor cells expression), showed PD-L1 (clone number 28-8) expressed in 52% (69/133) of GBMs (see **Figure 1**).

4.3 Prognostic value of PD-L1 in GBM patients

Many studies have investigated the association between PD-L1 expression levels and the prognosis of GBM patients. But the results from different studies are non-conclusive. Nduom et al. [43] discovered that positive PD-L1 expression was associated with a poor prognosis, though this result has limited significance. Two recent studies have suggested that positive PD-L1 immunostaining in human GBM tissue means a poor prognosis [44, 45]. However, Berghoff et al. proposed the PD-L1 was not a negative predictor of survival [41], and Lee et al. [46] found the PD-L1 expression did not appear to be an independent factor for unfavorable prognosis according to multivariate analysis.

Efforts aimed at inhibiting the PD-1/PDL1 pathway have shown more promising results. In a preclinical study using the GL261 glioma mouse model, combination of anti-PD-1 antibodies and radiotherapy doubled median survival and elicited long-term survival in 15–40% of mice compared with either treatment alone [34]. Clinically, pembrolizumab, a PD-L1 antibody has been approved by the FDA, to apply in the treatment of metastatic melanoma and NSCLC. In GBM, nivolumab, another PD-1 antibody, developed for GBM patients is being tested with two clinical trials [34].

A randomized Phase III study aimed at testing nivolumab versus bevacizumab in recurrent GBM patients will also test combination therapy of nivolumab and ipilimumab. Another two Phase I/II trials will analyze the effectiveness of combinatorial pembrolizumab and bevacizumab, and combinatorial pembrolizumab with MRI-guided laser ablation in recurrent GBM patients. In addition, MED14736, a humanized PD-L1 mAb, is currently being tested in clinical trials for GBM patients combined with radiotherapy and bevacizumab [34].

Currently, immunological checkpoint inhibitor drugs associated with PD-L1 for the treatment of glioblastoma are undergoing relevant clinical trials. Nivolumab is a fully humanized IgG4 subtype programmed death-1 (PD-1) immune checkpoint inhibitor antibody that binds with high affinity to PD-1 receptors on T cells and blocks their interaction with PD-L1 and restores T-cell antitumor function. There are several clinical trials of nivolumab for GBMs. The first large-scale randomized clinical trial of Checkmate 143(NCT 02017717) evaluated the safety and efficacy

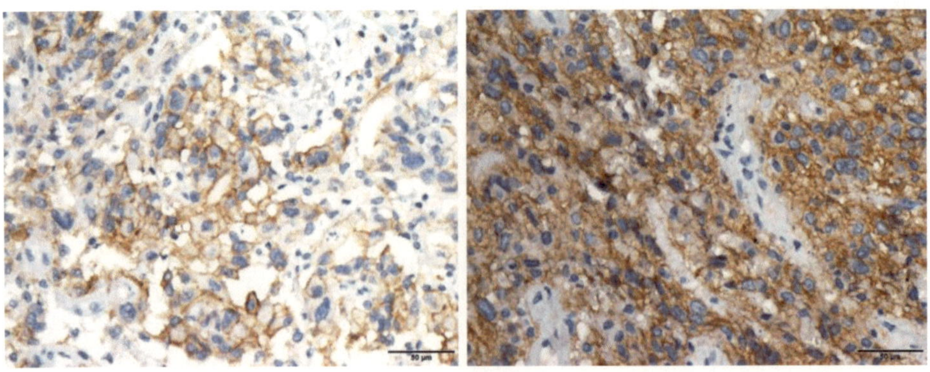

Figure 1.
The positive staining of PD-L1 in tumor cells by immunohistochemical stain. The brown color of the glioma cell membrane indicates the positive staining.

of nivolumab in GBM patients. In addition, the trial included a study comparing nivolumab monotherapy with bevacizumab in patients with recurrent GBM [47]. However, in the third phase of the clinical trial, 369 patients with first recurrence of GBM were recruited and it was found that nivolumab failed to prolong OS in patients compared with bevacizumab [48].

Pembrolizumab is another humanized monoclonal IgG4 anti-PD-1 antibody. Pembrolizumab was evaluated in 29 patients with high-grade malignant gliomas, including overall response rate (ORR) on contrast MRI, characterizing toxicities, progression-free survival (PFS), and overall survival (OS) [49]. Another trial about pembrolizumab showed that this drug is well tolerated, but the anti-PD-1 monotherapy was not effective for most GBM patients [50, 51].

In addition, other PD-L1 immune checkpoint inhibitor drugs for GBM that are being studied include durvalumab, atezolizumab, pidilizumab, and so on. Durvalumab is a fully humanized immunoglobulin G1k monoclonal antibody that blocks the binding of PD-L1 to PD-1 and CD80, thereby enhancing the identification and killing of tumor cells by T cells. Atezolizumab is a humanized immunoglobulin G1 (IgG1) monoclonal antibody directly targeting PD-L1. It prevents the interaction of PD-L1 with the receptors PD-1 and B7.1 by binding to L1. Currently, three open clinical trials (NCT 01375842, NCT02458638, and NCT03174197) are investigating atezolizumab in GBM patients. Pidilizumab is a humanized immunoglobulin (Ig) G1 monoclonal antibody directed against human PD-1 to block the combination between PD-1 and its ligands, PD-L1 and PD-L2. NCT01952769 is an ongoing clinical trial evaluating pidilizumab for GBM [52].

In future, besides PD-L1, more immune checkpoint inhibitors will be put into clinical trials to target this highly malignant brain tumor in future. Overall, the combination of various immune checkpoint modulators has shown promising effectiveness in the treatment of some solid tumors. The application of combinatorial checkpoint modulators in GBM and other tumors therefore requires further investigation into the interplay of co-stimulatory and coinhibitory molecules [34].

5. Conclusion

Although still in its infancy, immunotherapy for cancers has already shown significant effect against some types of malignancy, such as melanoma and lung cancer. Current open clinical trials of immunotherapy for GBM predominantly focus on dendritic cell (DC) vaccines and antibodies targeting immunosuppressive checkpoints have achieved promising immune activity and clinical responses. However, durable and sustained response remains rare, highlighting the need for novel promising approaches including gene therapy and combinatorial immunotherapeutic treatment [12].

Current obstacles for immune therapy for GBM lie in: (1) finding drugs to penetrate the BBB; (2) identifying specific, suitable, and immunogenic tumor antigens; and (3) identifying appropriate pre- and post-therapeutic biomarkers to reliably evaluate the treatment effect [34]. Additional research is necessary in the future to overcome those difficulties and identify a good treatment option or options for patients with GBM.

Author details

Wan-Ming Hu[1], Frank Y. Shan[2*], Sanjib Mukherjee[2], Danijela Levacic[2] and Jason H. Huang[2]

1 Department of Pathology, Sun Yat-sen University Cancer Center, Guangzhou, P.R. China

2 Department of Neurosurgery and Cancer Center, Baylor Scott and White Health, College of Medicine, Texas A&M University, Texas, USA

*Address all correspondence to: yshan918@gmail.com

References

[1] Tivnan A, Heilinger T, Lavelle EC, Prehn JH. Advances in immunotherapy for the treatment of glioblastoma. Journal of Neuro-Oncology. 2017;**131**(1):1-9

[2] Choi BD, Maus MV, June CH, Sampson JH. Immunotherapy for glioblastoma: Adoptive T-cell strategies. Clinical Cancer Research. 2019;**25**(7):2042-2048

[3] Palma L, Di Lorenzo N, Guidetti B. Lymphocytic infiltrates in primary glioblastomas and recidivous gliomas. Incidence, fate, and relevance to prognosis in 228 operated cases. Journal of Neurosurgery. 1978;**49**(6):854-861

[4] Brooks WH, Markesbery WR, Gupta GD, Roszman TL. Relationship of lymphocyte invasion and survival of brain tumor patients. Annals of Neurology. 1978;**4**(3):219-224

[5] Woroniecka KI, Rhodin KE, Chongsathidkiet P, Keith KA, Fecci PE. T-cell dysfunction in glioblastoma: Applying a new framework. Clinical Cancer Research. 2018;**24**(16):3792-3802

[6] Bielamowicz K, Fousek K, Byrd TT, Samaha H, Mukherjee M, Aware N, et al. Trivalent CAR T cells overcome interpatient antigenic variability in glioblastoma. Neuro-Oncology. 2018;**20**(4):506-518

[7] O'Rourke DM, Nasrallah MP, Desai A, Melenhorst JJ, Mansfield K, Morrissette J, et al. A single dose of peripherally infused EGFRvIII-directed CAR T cells mediates antigen loss and induces adaptive resistance in patients with recurrent glioblastoma. Science Translational Medicine. 2017;**9**(399)

[8] Brown CE, Badie B, Barish ME, Weng L, Ostberg JR, Chang WC, et al. Bioactivity and safety of IL13Ralpha2-redirected chimeric antigen receptor CD8+ T cells in patients with recurrent glioblastoma. Clinical Cancer Research. 2015;**21**(18):4062-4072

[9] Ahmed N, Brawley V, Hegde M, Bielamowicz K, Kalra M, Landi D, et al. HER2-specific chimeric antigen receptor-modified virus-specific T cells for progressive glioblastoma: A phase 1 dose-escalation trial. JAMA Oncology. 2017;**3**(8):1094-1101

[10] Yeku OO, Purdon TJ, Koneru M, Spriggs D, Brentjens RJ. Armored CAR T cells enhance antitumor efficacy and overcome the tumor microenvironment. Scientific Reports. 2017;**7**(1):10541

[11] Farber SH, Elsamadicy AA, Atik AF, Suryadevara CM, Chongsathidkiet P, Fecci PE, et al. The Safety of available immunotherapy for the treatment of glioblastoma. Expert Opinion on Drug Safety. 2017;**16**(3):277-287

[12] Huang B, Zhang H, Gu L, Ye B, Jian Z, Stary C, et al. Advances in immunotherapy for glioblastoma multiforme. Journal of Immunology Research. 2017;**2017**:3597613

[13] Hamblett KJ, Kozlosky CJ, Siu S, Chang WS, Liu H, Foltz IN, et al. AMG 595, an anti-EGFRvIII antibody-drug conjugate, induces potent antitumor activity against EGFRvIII-expressing glioblastoma. Molecular Cancer Therapeutics. 2015;**14**(7):1614-1624

[14] Keller S, Schmidt M. EGFR and EGFRvIII promote angiogenesis and cell invasion in glioblastoma: Combination therapies for an effective treatment. International Journal of Molecular Sciences. 2017;**18**(6):1295

[15] Ekstrand AJ, Sugawa N, James CD, Collins VP. Amplified and rearranged epidermal growth factor receptor genes

in human glioblastomas reveal deletions of sequences encoding portions of the N- and/or C-terminal tails. Proceedings of the National Academy of Sciences of the United States of America. 1992;**89**(10):4309-4313

[16] Malden LT, Novak U, Kaye AH, Burgess AW. Selective amplification of the cytoplasmic domain of the epidermal growth factor receptor gene in glioblastoma multiforme. Cancer Research. 1988;**48**(10):2711-2714

[17] Sugawa N, Ekstrand AJ, James CD, Collins VP. Identical splicing of aberrant epidermal growth factor receptor transcripts from amplified rearranged genes in human glioblastomas. Proceedings of the National Academy of Sciences of the United States of America. 1990;**87**(21):8602-8606

[18] Shinojima N, Tada K, Shiraishi S, Kamiryo T, Kochi M, Nakamura H, et al. Prognostic value of epidermal growth factor receptor in patients with glioblastoma multiforme. Cancer Research. 2003;**63**(20):6962-6970

[19] Donson AM, Addo-Yobo SO, Handler MH, Gore L, Foreman NK. MGMT promoter methylation correlates with survival benefit and sensitivity to temozolomide in pediatric glioblastoma. Pediatric Blood & Cancer. 2007;**48**(4):403-407

[20] Kreth S, Limbeck E, Hinske LC, Schutz SV, Thon N, Hoefig K, et al. In human glioblastomas transcript elongation by alternative polyadenylation and miRNA targeting is a potent mechanism of MGMT silencing. Acta Neuropathologica. 2013;**125**(5):671-681

[21] Wikstrand CJ, Hale LP, Batra SK, Hill ML, Humphrey PA, Kurpad SN, et al. Monoclonal antibodies against EGFRvIII are tumor specific and react with breast and lung carcinomas and malignant gliomas. Cancer Research. 1995;**55**(14):3140-3148

[22] Nishikawa R, Ji XD, Harmon RC, Lazar CS, Gill GN, Cavenee WK, et al. A mutant epidermal growth factor receptor common in human glioma confers enhanced tumorigenicity. Proceedings of the National Academy of Sciences of the United States of America. 1994;**91**(16):7727-7731

[23] Moscatello DK, Holgado-Madruga M, Godwin AK, Ramirez G, Gunn G, Zoltick PW, et al. Frequent expression of a mutant epidermal growth factor receptor in multiple human tumors. Cancer Research. 1995;**55**(23):5536-5539

[24] Olapade-Olaopa EO, Moscatello DK, MacKay EH, Horsburgh T, Sandhu DP, Terry TR, et al. Evidence for the differential expression of a variant EGF receptor protein in human prostate cancer. British Journal of Cancer. 2000;**82**(1):186-194

[25] Viana-Pereira M, Lopes JM, Little S, Milanezi F, Basto D, Pardal F, et al. Analysis of EGFR overexpression, EGFR gene amplification and the EGFRvIII mutation in Portuguese high-grade gliomas. Anticancer Research. 2008;**28**(2A):913-920

[26] Rosenthal M, Curry R, Reardon DA, Rasmussen E, Upreti VV, Damore MA, et al. Safety, tolerability, and pharmacokinetics of anti-EGFRvIII antibody-drug conjugate AMG 595 in patients with recurrent malignant glioma expressing EGFRvIII. Cancer Chemotherapy and Pharmacology. 2019;**84**(2):327-336

[27] Gan HK, Cvrljevic AN, Johns TG. The epidermal growth factor receptor variant III (EGFRvIII): Where wild things are altered. The FEBS Journal. 2013;**280**(21):5350-5370

[28] Batra SK, Castelino-Prabhu S, Wikstrand CJ, Zhu X, Humphrey PA, Friedman HS, et al. Epidermal growth factor ligand-independent, unregulated, cell-transforming potential of a naturally occurring human mutant EGFRvIII gene. Cell Growth & Differentiation. 1995;**6**(10):1251-1259

[29] Nagane M, Coufal F, Lin H, Bogler O, Cavenee WK, Huang HJ. A common mutant epidermal growth factor receptor confers enhanced tumorigenicity on human glioblastoma cells by increasing proliferation and reducing apoptosis. Cancer Research. 1996;**56**(21):5079-5086

[30] Narita Y, Nagane M, Mishima K, Huang HJ, Furnari FB, Cavenee WK. Mutant epidermal growth factor receptor signaling down-regulates p27 through activation of the phosphatidylinositol 3-kinase/Akt pathway in glioblastomas. Cancer Research. 2002;**62**(22):6764-6769

[31] Lal A, Glazer CA, Martinson HM, Friedman HS, Archer GE, Sampson JH, et al. Mutant epidermal growth factor receptor up-regulates molecular effectors of tumor invasion. Cancer Research. 2002;**62**(12):3335-3339

[32] Phillips AC, Boghaert ER, Vaidya KS, Mitten MJ, Norvell S, Falls HD, et al. ABT-414, an antibody-drug conjugate targeting a tumor-selective EGFR epitope. Molecular Cancer Therapeutics. 2016;**15**(4):661-669

[33] Balkwill F, Mantovani A. Inflammation and cancer: Back to Virchow? Lancet. 2001;**357**(9255):539-545

[34] Bloch O, Crane CA, Kaur R, Safaee M, Rutkowski MJ, Parsa AT. Gliomas promote immunosuppression through induction of B7-H1 expression in tumor-associated macrophages. Clinical Cancer Research. 2013;**19**(12):3165-3175

[35] Dong H, Strome SE, Salomao DR, Tamura H, Hirano F, Flies DB, et al. Tumor-associated B7-H1 promotes T-cell apoptosis: A potential mechanism of immune evasion. Nature Medicine. 2002;**8**(8):793-800

[36] Intlekofer AM, Thompson CB. At the bench: Preclinical rationale for CTLA-4 and PD-1 blockade as cancer immunotherapy. Journal of Leukocyte Biology. 2013;**94**(1):25-39

[37] Dong H, Zhu G, Tamada K, Chen L. B7-H1, a third member of the B7 family, co-stimulates T-cell proliferation and interleukin-10 secretion. Nature Medicine. 1999;**5**(12):1365-1369

[38] Stupp R, Hegi ME, Mason WP, van den Bent MJ, Taphoorn MJ, Janzer RC, et al. Effects of radiotherapy with concomitant and adjuvant temozolomide versus radiotherapy alone on survival in glioblastoma in a randomised phase III study: 5-year analysis of the EORTC-NCIC trial. The Lancet Oncology. 2009;**10**(5):459-466

[39] Parsa AT, Waldron JS, Panner A, Crane CA, Parney IF, Barry JJ, et al. Loss of tumor suppressor PTEN function increases B7-H1 expression and immunoresistance in glioma. Nature Medicine. 2007;**13**(1):84-88

[40] Liu Y, Carlsson R, Ambjorn M, Hasan M, Badn W, Darabi A, et al. PD-L1 expression by neurons nearby tumors indicates better prognosis in glioblastoma patients. The Journal of Neuroscience. 2013;**33**(35):14231-14245

[41] Berghoff AS, Kiesel B, Widhalm G, Rajky O, Ricken G, Wohrer A, et al. Programmed death ligand 1 expression and tumor-infiltrating lymphocytes in glioblastoma. Neuro-Oncology. 2015;**17**(8):1064-1075

[42] Xiu J, Piccioni D, Juarez T, Pingle SC, Hu J, Rudnick J, et al.

Multi-platform molecular profiling of a large cohort of glioblastomas reveals potential therapeutic strategies. Oncotarget. 2016;7(16):21556-21569

[43] Nduom EK, Wei J, Yaghi NK, Huang N, Kong LY, Gabrusiewicz K, et al. PD-L1 expression and prognostic impact in glioblastoma. Neuro-Oncology. 2016;**18**(2):195-205

[44] Han J, Hong Y, Lee YS. PD-L1 expression and combined status of PD-L1/PD-1-positive tumor infiltrating mononuclear cell density predict prognosis in glioblastoma patients. Journal of Pathology and Translational Medicine. 2017;**51**(1):40-48

[45] Zeng J, Zhang XK, Chen HD, Zhong ZH, Wu QL, Lin SX. Expression of programmed cell death-ligand 1 and its correlation with clinical outcomes in gliomas. Oncotarget. 2016;7(8):8944-8955

[46] Lee KS, Lee K, Yun S, Moon S, Park Y, Han JH, et al. Prognostic relevance of programmed cell death ligand 1 expression in glioblastoma. Journal of Neuro-Oncology. 2018;**136**(3):453-461

Abedalthagafi M, Barakeh D, Foshay KM. Immunogenetics of glioblastoma: The future of personalized patient management. NPJ Precision Oncology. 2018;**2**:27

[47] Omuro A, Vlahovic G, Lim M, Sahebjam S, Baehring J, Cloughesy T, et al. Nivolumab with or without ipilimumab in patients with recurrent glioblastoma: Results from exploratory phase I cohorts of CheckMate 143. Neuro-Oncology. 2018;**20**(5):674-686

[48] Reiss SN, Yerram P, Modelevsky L, Grommes C. Retrospective review of safety and efficacy of programmed cell death-1 inhibitors in refractory high grade gliomas. Journal for Immunotherapy of Cancer. 2017;5(1):99

[49] Majd N, de Groot J. Challenges and strategies for successful clinical development of immune checkpoint inhibitors in glioblastoma. Expert Opinion on Pharmacotherapy. 2019;**20**(13):1609-1624

[50] Harrison RA, Anderson MD, Cachia D, Kamiya-Matsuoka C, Weathers SS, O'Brien BJ, et al. Clinical trial participation of patients with glioblastoma at The University of Texas MD Anderson Cancer Center. European Journal of Cancer. 2019;**112**:83-93

[51] Caccese M, Indraccolo S, Zagonel V, Lombardi G. PD-1/PD-L1 immune-checkpoint inhibitors in glioblastoma: A concise review. Critical Reviews in Oncology/Hematology. 2019;**135**:128-134